The Art and Science of Intermittent Fasting For Women

How to Achieve Lasting Weight Loss, A Lean Body, Keep Hormones in Balance and Live A Healthy Lifestyle

Jamie Connor

The following eBook is produced below with the goal of providing information that is as accurate and reliable as possible. Regardless, purchasing this Book can be seen as consent to the fact that both the publisher and the author of this book are in no way experts on the topics discussed within and that any recommendations or suggestions that are made herein are for entertainment purposes only. Professionals should be consulted as needed prior to undertaking any of the action endorsed herein.

This declaration is deemed fair and valid by both the American Bar Association and the Committee of Publishers Association and is legally binding throughout the United States.

Furthermore, the transmission, duplication or reproduction of any of the following work including specific information will be considered an illegal act irrespective of if it is done electronically or in print. This extends to creating a secondary or tertiary copy of the work or a recorded copy and is only allowed with express written consent from the Publisher. All additional rights reserved.

Table of Contents

Chapter 1: Intermittent Fasting...What Is It?

Fad diets and ridiculous weight loss programs have always plagued our society, but in today's digital age the problem has gotten much, much worse. This age of mass information sharing has positively impacted the world in many ways, but there are also some downsides. Anecdotal claims and extreme diets are now heavily promoted with little to no scientific basis. In this book we are going to use scientific and academic based research to discuss everything you need to know about Intermittent fasting as a woman. Once you have the knowledge to fully understand what you are doing and how it is affecting your body, you will then have to implement this knowledge into your real life. Doing this takes time, patience, and effort. This whole process of Learning something new and creating a new life for yourself should be treated as an art form, because it is.

Fasting has been practiced for centuries around the globe for a wide variety of cultural, religious, and biologically beneficial ways. It actually developed all over the world centuries ago in completely separated groups of people. In ancient Greece, fasting was used as a way of preparing for spiritual events. Great philosophers like Pythagoras used fasting as a way for them to obtain dreams and visions. [14] For thousands of years, Muslims have been fasting during their holy month of Ramadan, every day, from sunrise to sunset.

There have been commonalities in the way fasting is viewed over countless cultures, one, in particular, are its possible biological benefits. In the mid-1800s we see an early academic documentation or statement of this in E.H *Dewey's "The True Science of Living."* He believed that every disease that humans are afflicted with in one way or another was linked to "habitual eating in excess." [14] Later on in the early to mid-1900s, a lot more medical research was done on fasting. In 1915 actually, fasting was a widely used method to treat obesity and in a particular instance, a group of doctors and associates placed obese individuals on prolonged fasting regimens with the longest lasting 382 days! [14] Yes, that was an obese man who consequently lost 276 pounds from that year and a bit, but it really shows you what the human body can do.

We will start by diving into the science of fasting and how intermittent fasting can affect you as a woman. We will then debunk some common myths you may have heard about intermittent fasting or just fasting in general, followed by the ways you can practice and implement it into your life.

Those doctors in 1915 were not just recommending fasting. They were starving their patients. Nowadays, we like to be a bit more methodical. Controlled fasting has shown its benefits when executed properly in many individuals, as you will soon see. Fasting has gained a bad rep in some cases due to individuals who really just have not yet educated themselves on yes the benefits, but also the risks. So how do we fast methodically? We can do this through something called *Intermittent Fasting (IF)*.

What is **Intermittent Fasting**? No, it is not some crash diet or some extreme method of losing weight. The media has bombarded us with enough of those. Intermittent fasting is a methodical practice with ancient ties that, when done right, brings a wide variety of benefits to your physical and psychological well-being. Intermittent fasting is a time-restricted eating method, or metabolic exercise, where an individual will fast typically periodically, with many variations, multiple times a week. It is important to note that while IF is a good way to lose weight in a healthy way when executed properly, it is also an effective way of preventing future bad weight gain. Practicing these methods and implementing them into your life can have lasting benefits, not just a quick fix followed by a quick break.

It's not a pure coincidence most of us are taught at a very young age that we need to consume three square meals a day, with breakfast being the most important. Not only is this system of eating perfect for keeping the consumer, that's you, in a fed state. This increases the chance dramatically that you will need more food at predictable times. Companies like Kellogg's for example have wildly benefitted from the marketing to everyone that "breakfast should never be missed." This kind of thing may sound scary because so many of us are used to eating many small meals throughout the day in order to keep our metabolism up. Eating like this, however, can actually have dangerous effects on your overall health due to consistently elevated levels of insulin. This pancreas-produced hormone helps regulate the levels of glucose. As a woman, you will want to know how intermittent fasting will affect your hormones that we will cover in a later chapter. In a healthy human body, the amount of glucose in your blood will rise when you eat any food and your pancreas will release insulin in order to guide the glucose into cells and thus use it. If you have extra insulin, it can guide the glucose into muscle or fat cells to store for later. With higher levels of insulin your bodies *"fat burning process"* shuts off and your body starts to break down the energy from your last meal instead.

These are key traits of two different and opposing states the human body transitions between; a **fed state** and a **fasted state**. [1]

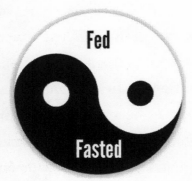

In a **fed state**, your body will use the glucose from your last meal to provide energy for your body. This will not only leave previously stored energy in fat cells but also actually send even more glucose for storage to those same cells. However, why would someone be hungry if they have previously stored energy? This is because their body has been in a fed state far too long. This can have drastic changes to anyone on a cellular level. In a cell, there are basic common structures tasked with specific duties for the proper functioning of that cell. One of these structures is called the mitochondria, also known as the powerhouse of the cell. When your insulin guides glucose into cells, your mitochondria are what break it down into energy. They also break down fat into energy, and they can have a preference. Consistently being in a fed state with spikes and drops of insulin and glucose levels creates a systematic preference within the mitochondria. Slowly, your mitochondria increase the glucose pathways whilst reducing the number of fat burning pathways. Eventually, every time glucose levels decrease in your body the mitochondria will starve for more. [1] You can then find your self-trapped in an addiction like cycle where your body depends on more glucose every few hours, all while continually storing, not using, the excess energy in your cells.

In a **fasted state,** however, your body will use a lot more fat-burning pathways due to low levels of insulin and glucose. First, the energy in your liver, called Glycogen is the most easily accessible and used. Then the energy you have previously stored in your fat cells is what will be used for your body to function. On the other hand, if you have been in a fed state for far too long, adapting your body back to fat usage will need to be a purposeful process. Meaning you will have to take actions yourself to allow your body to increase slowly the number of fat burning pathways you have in your mitochondria. A perfect method for this is *intermittent fasting*. Remember, however, it's a metabolic exercise that takes time and effort to get right.

When your metabolic processes and body's energy are primarily using fat stores as energy, this is called **ketosis. This is not to be confused with ketoacidosis;** a term commonly used with individuals who are type I diabetics. For them, instead of just running on fat stores when they are in a fasted state, they can eat a whole meal and their body will not produce the insulin needed to digest the energy, it will still keep running on fat stores.

As simply put before, the transition between a fed state and fasted state is a process. George Cahill, an American scientist who significantly contributed to the advancement of Diabetes research, found that this transition actually happens in 5 different stages.[4] George Cahill documented this information while he studied how starvation affected metabolism. [4]

During *intermittent fasting*, the most widely used methods will only have you in stage 1 and stage 2. Stage 3 can only occur beyond 16 hours of fasting. This would be a danger zone. Part of the point of purposefully fasting periodically is to control how the body uses previously stored energy, not to starve yourself into losing weight and possibly damaging hormonal function.

Phase I is Feeding: When we eat any food, our blood sugar (glucose levels) will rise. Following this, our insulin levels will rise in order to use the glucose for instant energy and/or store excess in fat cells or as glycogen in the liver.

Phase II is the Post Absorptive Stage: This is where the glycogen that has been previously stored in your liver is starting to be used. Following this, the energy stored in fat cells will be used.

Origin of Blood Glucose	Stage 1 of Fasting Transition	Stage 2 of Fasting Transition	Stage 3 of Fasting Transition
Tissues Using Glucose	All	Everything except for the liver, muscles, and lower levels of adipose tissues	Everything except for the liver, muscles, and significantly diminished levels of adipose tissues
Fuel of Brain	Glucose	Glucose	Glucose

Chapter 2: How Intermittent Fasting Benefits Your Health

Right now, we have a global epidemic of obesity and diabetes plaguing our society physically, emotionally and financially. In fact, approximately 2.8 million people globally die every year to obesity-related illnesses according to the WHO. Not only does this mean an early grave, but it can also mean a lifelong struggle and disability. Issues like diabetes, ischemic heart disease, certain cancers, and an array of health problems can all be attributed to Obesity. (5) Some unfortunate individuals are born with predispositions to these diseases; however, a vast majority can be attributed to lifelong eating habits. Eating highly processed foods full of **saturated fat** and **LDL Cholesterol** throughout the entire day maintaining your body's fed state is a key contributor to developing obesity. If you eat like this, not only are you forming a mitochondrial addiction as your insulin levels constantly spike throughout the day, but you are accompanying that with artery clogging, brain damaging and cancer-causing substances.

So how does Intermittent fasting help with all of this? Firstly, we will cover the physical health benefits then move on to the beneficial mental results you can achieve from it. These are things such as undergoing healthy weight loss. Let us start with the metabolic disease Diabetes. Someone has Diabetes when their body does not produce enough or any insulin and/or when their body's cells do not know how to react to insulin. This inadequacy of insulin can leave individuals with dangerously high glucose levels in their blood. Intermittent fasting lets you better control insulin levels actually. *The World Journal of Diabetes* found that intermittent fasting on a regular basis helped reduce post-meal glucose spikes. Individuals with diabetes, however, should take extra precautions to maintain more stable glucose levels, nutrition and maintaining caloric sufficiency will be covered in a later chapter.

Healthy Weight Loss

One of the most commonly known benefits from intermittent fasting is the **healthy weight loss**. With this weight loss also comes improvements to your cardiovascular health and your gut health. The weight loss will almost be immediate once you start practicing a periodic fasting regimen due to the inevitable lower caloric intake. We will discuss more about caloric intake later on. In a systematic review of 40 unique intermittent fasting studies, the average weight loss recorded was 7-11 pounds over 10 weeks. [2] Take note that the participants ranged in size from lean to obese. Leaner individuals will typically experience a less drastic weight loss compared to their larger counterparts. Losing excess weight comes with more benefits for your cardiovascular system. Things like hypertension, which are three times more prevalent in obese individuals, and congestive heart failure have been found to have a direct correlation with being overweight and obese.

According to the American Heart Association, for patients experiencing these problems, "reductions in weight dramatically improve ventricular function and oxygenation." However, it is not just the heart; your gut will benefit too. Our gut is actually much more complex than you may assume. In every human gut, there live thousands of species like bacteria, viruses, fungi, and amoebae. These microbes can actually alter how we metabolize our foods, and even alter how they tell our body when it should feel hungry. These complex communities of microbes change over time and can be directly affected by the environment they are subject to. In 2017, a study in cell metabolism found that there was an increase in the fermentation products *acetate and lactate* that help fat cells produce more mitochondria. Increased mitochondria of these cells mean stored fat is being used as energy more than before. An almost guaranteed benefit you can get from intermittent fasting is weight loss and thus significantly reducing your risk to any of this issue and ailments.

Healthy Skin

Then there is the outside of your body, the part that everybody sees every day, your skin. Your skin can be a clear indicator of how your body is in that moment and it can reflect how it has been treated. Constantly being in a fed state can put a lot of stress on your body as it is always focused on digesting your last meal. Stress can represent itself in so many ways including blotchy skin, redness, inflammation, and acne. Coupled with a diet high in saturated fat and processed oils, you would be lucky not to show any signs. Intermittent fasting not only allows your body to completely digest food then focus on functioning optimally but also typically increases the amount of water you will drink. Women need more water as is due to the estrogen and progesterone that lowers blood plasma volumes, and in turn, can bring on quicker fatigue or dehydration. While intermittent fasting, you will be drinking significantly more water throughout the week which comes with its own plethora of benefits for the skin and rest of your body.

When your body is focusing on digesting in a fed state, it is also in a **parasympathetic state** through your automatic nervous system (ANS). Your ANS has two states as well, sympathetic and parasympathetic. The sympathetic nervous

19

system is active when you are in "fight or flight" mode, basically, anytime you are actively using your skeletal muscles. The parasympathetic state is when you are in a "rest and digest" mode and your body's energy is going towards the internal functioning of digestive organs. Staying a Fed and Parasympathetic state continuously can lead to negative effects on your mood, motivation, brain health, and sleep. Studies done by the University of Virginia concluded that consistent IF [might] improve cognitive functions and brain structures.

Better Sleep

Intermittent fasting can also improve your sleeping patterns. However, have you ever actually tried sleeping on an empty stomach? It is hard, isn't it? That is because most of us are so used to being in that fed state, basically having a full stomach, and our systems are literally depending on more energy from food entering the body. However, after the initial adjustment period, fasting has shown to be able to improve sleep quality in a variety of studies. One group of researchers and experts in particular in the Dept. of Internal Medicine at Kliniken Essen Mitte in Germany conducted an open pilot study that was able to come to this conclusion disturbances in sleeping patterns are lowered hence the night time rests are peaceful and uninterrupted. The one-week long fasting aided in this and in effect, the energy levels and strength of these individuals belonging to normal BMI levels are better more than ever in their day-to-day activities. What is particularly useful about this study is that 92% of the test subjects were women. They measured sleep patterns of these women using polysomnography.

Polysomnography is a widely used method of diagnosing sleep disorders and monitoring sleep patterns. It is done by measuring the brain waves, oxygen levels, eye, and facial twitching, the heartbeat, breathing patterns, and any muscle movements of the subject as they sleep. Once you get yourself over the adjustment period, you can expect to see improvements in your morning mood and energy. It is important to note their findings on obese subjects too. It's one theory that the practice of periodic or intermittent fasting triggered both weight loss, reduced stress on the body from constantly combating glucose spikes, and allowed the individuals parasympathetic nervous system to diet all functions to obtaining adequate rest for the body, as opposed to digesting food and adjust blood sugar levels during their sleep.

Intermittent fasting comes with this array of benefits and reduces risk to so many preventable diseases, but it is not to be taken lightly. If done wrong you can endanger yourself, so you have to take the right precautions when deciding to live this way. You should consider all personal circumstances too. Nevertheless, if you think you're ready, it is time to pick a method and make it yours! For a quick reference of some the benefits intermittent fasting can bring you, check out the graphic on the next page.

Which Women Should Avoid or Be Extra Cautious About Intermittent Fasting?

Depending on what stage of life you are in and your special circumstances, any form of intermittent fasting might not be for you. Any form of fasting is not recommended if you are breastfeeding or pregnant. When you are pregnant, the food you will be consuming is for two individuals and fasting can cause a high risk for potential harm to the fetus. Healthy fetal development depends on a wide range of hormones and their processes can heavily depend on the functioning of the parts of your brain important for hormones. These hormonal glands are going to be affected directly during a fast due to the inevitably lower insulin levels you will have. Intermittent fasting can affect every woman differently but the adverse short-term effects are relatively benign. When you are pregnant, those short-term adverse effects can be life-threatening for the fetus and potentially permanently damaging.

Women who are diabetic or have previously diagnosed with metabolic syndrome will have to take extra care when intermittent fasting. Diseases like metabolic syndrome, when your body's metabolism is messed up in one way or another, are rooted in how insulin acts in your body and insulin is the most important hormone affected by any fasting regimen.

Benefits of Intermittent Fasting for Women (Quick Guide)

Diabetes Management

Intermittent fasting allows you to better control your insulin levels and reduce the traditional post meal spike of glucose

Sleep Like a Baby

Many studies have shown that even professional athletes can perform optimally during long periods of fasting

Let them Grow

Studies show that during periods of fasting, the microbes of your gut produce more mitochondria

Lose some excess weight

Intermittent fasting decreases your caloric intake and emphasis the use of stored fat as energy instead of glucose

Reduced Risk of Cancer

A lower intake of calories while practicing IF has shown a significantly reduced risk to obesity/diet related

Happy Girl

Allowing your body to stay in a fasted state can divert your bodies energy towards optimal dopamine production

Beautiful Skin

Not only will you be drinking more water and hydrating your skin but the reduced stress helps combat breakouts

Cardiovascular Health

Partially due to the inevitable weight loss, your risk for congestive heart failure or hypertension are reduced dramatically

Chapter 3: As a Woman, What Can You Expect from Your Hormones in Reaction to Intermittent Fasting?

Hormones, they make us who we are even though they may sometimes portray us as people we are not. Hormones in the human body have a massive impact on every function you can think of. This is especially true for women. I say this because your caloric and nutritional intake can have direct influences on the hormones that are involved with important processes such as ovulation. Some women have reported missing periods, have developed metabolic stress issues, and even early onset menopause. [6]

This is why it is so important to pick methodically your method or variation of intermittent fasting and plans to see what you, as a unique individual, will need. One that will certainly be of interest to you is the Crescendo fasting method, which we will dive into in Chapter 5. Women's bodies are much more sensitive to hormonal imbalances for a number of reasons.

(6) This is not a negative thing; no this is Mother Nature just doing her work to protect the existence of future children. When your body feels it is entering a state of starvation, a hormonal process starts.

First, you should know how your hormones work. In both women and men, hormones are controlled by the cooperation of three endocrine glands. These are the hypothalamus, the pituitary gland, and the gonads. Your hypothalamus, your brain, will release a specific hormone that then creates a chain reaction of events throughout your body that ultimately effect two very important hormones. Estrogen and Progesterone are two very important hormones as I am sure you are aware. Both play vital roles in female development but also are required for producing a mature egg, AKA ovulation, as well as throughout actual pregnancy.

So how does fasting affect this process? Well, the GnRH that is released by your hypothalamus has actually shown evidence of being sensitive to environmental factors. If this were the case, then it would mess up the entire hormonal system if we were to shock it. At the same time, however, sensitivity would also vary from individual to individual and this could be a possible cause for the reported cases of missing periods and early onset menopause. Your thyroid is also a crucial part of hormonal processes, but we will be covering that in the Chapter 6 section 'Psychological Hunger vs. Physiological Hunger.'

Insulin Resistance

As you now know, your insulin is also another major hormone affected by intermittent fasting. You do this by regulating your intake of energy and thus your blood sugar. This is done methodically and periodically over time with the goal to **decrease your insulin resistance.** Insulin resistance makes it difficult or does not even allow our body cells to recognize or interact with insulin in the bloodstream. When we eat, the blood sugar rises, then insulin is released into our bloodstream except, when individuals who are insulin resistant get to this stage and their cells don't know what to do, the sugars you just ate are then stored as glycogen in the liver or muscle and fat cells.

So how does one develop insulin resistance? The main contributors to developing insulin resistance are excess belly fat, poor diet being overweight, a lack of exercise and physical activity, as well as smoking and skimping on sleep. You do not just develop insulin resistance after a binge weekend of Ben and Jerry's Sweet Chili Heat Doritos, Oreos, and Netflix (all of which are completely plant-based by the way). However, insulin resistance develops over a prolonged period of time. You will not even notice the problems consciously as the problem develops but your body will still be fighting back. As your cells become more and more resistant to the insulin, your pancreas will produce more. If nothing changes, the cells will become even more resistant and the pancreas will be forced to produce even more insulin. This is completely overworking the pancreatic cells in charge and eventually, you will start to see your average blood sugar rise. This is when there is a real alarm for concern because now you would be at risk of pre-diabetes or full-blown type 2 diabetes or even something called non-alcoholic fatty liver disease or NAFLD that in turn boosts your risk significantly for any other permanent liver damage and even a higher risk of heart disease. [19]

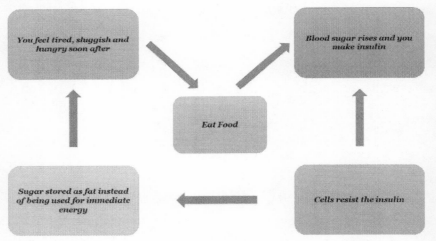

Insulin plays a vital role in women's bodily functions so you will want to make sure you are not experiencing any symptoms of insulin resistance before something more sinister develops. According to experts at the National Institute of Diabetes who studied pre-diabetes and insulin resistance, they found common symptoms that can help you identify possible problem trends early on. Some of the symptoms of insulin resistance developing are the following:

- High Blood Pressure and Sugar
- Large Waist
  - o For the average women, this is over 35 inches unless you are of Chinese, South Asian, or Japanese descent, then your number is 31.5 inches.
- Low Levels of Good Cholesterol (HDL)

Insulin resistance left ignored, can put you at a significantly higher risk to an array of diseases such as cancer of bladder, cervix, uterus, pancreas, and colon. (21)

Insulin Sensitivity

Part of the goal with intermittent fasting is to **increase your insulin sensitivity** by reducing the number and frequency of glucose spikes you have in a day. Women who are naturally insulin sensitive have an advantage because their bodies do not need as much insulin to regulate and direct glucose. Most women who are insulin sensitive actually acquired the trait through their genes but it is still possible to change if you were not born that way. Through exercise, sleeping patterns and especially diet we can gradually change for the better our insulin processes, just like our hormone process.

This is why nutrition will play a key part in practicing any method safely and properly. Nutrition can seem like a daunting subject with loads of information to take in but it really does not have to be. Find out in the next chapter.

Chapter 4: Nutrition and Intermittent Fasting

I like to think of nutrition as the process of obtaining the right quantity and quality of food in order to maintain a healthy body. It plays a key role in your body even before you are even born. Your mother's nutrition during, and possibly even before, affects how you as a fetus developed. Fast forward 9 months and the nutrition of your infancy and adolescence affected the way your brain, body, and hormonal processes developed. Up until this day, the trends in the food you eat on a daily basis will appear through their respective changes in your body. Considering this, there will be many things you should know about yourself when planning your own diet. Are you a diabetic? Do you have a preexisting thyroid issue? Are you celiac and thus gluten-free? However, before you plan, you should know the basics of how nutrition itself, how to calculate what you will need, how to track it on a daily basis or even just in general, and things that you should just stay away from.

Calories, protein, carbohydrates, fats, and vitamins/minerals, these are the six main nutrients you need to know in tracking your nutrition properly.

Calories

This is the single most important thing you need to consider during any type of diet. Calories are our way of measuring energy consumption from the foods we eat. Specifically, one calorie is what it takes to raise the temperature of a kg. of water by one degree Celsius. More calories equate to more energy consumed. Contrary to a myth, there are no foods "negative" in calories meaning there are no foods that will burn calories as you eat it. Yes, even celery, This may sound confusing but do not worry, you don't have to be aware of "thermic effects" at any time in your life. This is just to better help you understand how all foods you consume provide you energy in one way or another. Calories, and how many you consume compared to how many you burn, are also the basis of weight loss. A caloric surplus will generally lead to weight gain and a caloric deficit will typically lead to weight loss.

Calories are the **most important** thing to watch during any type of diet because if you consume enough calories, you more than likely consumed sufficient amounts of most of your required nutrients. As for weight loss, calories are also extremely important. You can attribute any weight gain to a caloric surplus, meaning you are consuming more calories than you are burning. The same goes for the other way, if you consume fewer calories than you burn you will be in a **caloric**

deficit, and thus lose weight. That is, with a reasonably diverse diet containing varieties of foods. Therefore, if you feel that tracking all your nutrients to be too much of an arduous task, you can just guide yourself towards a daily/weekly goal of a given number of calories, at least to start.

According to the US Department of Agriculture, women ages, 17-25 need approximately 2,000-2,400 calories, women who are between the age of between 26 and 50 will need approximately 1,800-2,200 calories per day and women above the age of 50 1,600-2,000 calories. Please note that they calculated these based on an estimated energy requirement and thus is a largely simplified representation of what the true values could be. For instance, they classify an active individual as someone who "[walks] 3 miles per day at 3 to 4 miles per hour," to do only 2 hours of light cardio per week this would be a near equivalent. It only takes 30 minutes of walking at a brisk pace, around 4mph, to burn 200 calories if you are a 175lb woman. This also a very basic estimation but it can give you an idea about the levels of energy expenditure in your daily activities or exercise.

Obviously, while you are intermittent fasting, you will lower your energy input significantly. This is the reason you need to pay extra attention to the calories you consume. Not all calories are the same and the food you consume will, in turn, bring you certain types of energy. The calories you get from a can of coke are approximately 142 calories but they bring virtually no nutritional qualities with them and just inject you with 39 grams of sugar. Consumption of these "empty" calories brings on artificial sensations of satiety along with stimulating and addictive high-fructose corn syrup, which in turn adds to the already spiking glucose levels of the average all-day diet. On the other hand, 142 calories of calories of unsweetened soymilk would give you approximately 14 grams of protein, 4 grams of healthy fats, zero cholesterol, low in sodium and all with only 2 grams of sugar.

The number of calories you will need as an individual will depend on a variety of factors: your height, weight, metabolic tendencies, and most importantly your lifestyle.

Gender	Age (Years)	Physical Activity		
		Sedentary	Moderately Active	Active
Female	2 - 3	1000 - 1200	1000 - 1400	1000 - 1400
	4 - 8	1200 - 1400	1400 - 1600	1400 - 1800
	9 - 13	1400 - 1600	1600 - 2000	1800 - 2200
	14 - 18	1800	2000	2400
	19 - 30	1800 - 2000	2000 - 2200	2400
	31 - 50	1800	2000	2200
	51 +	1600	1800	2000 - 2200

Protein

Protein is the holy grail of muscle building and athlete performance. Protein molecules are also known as polypeptides. These are composed over 20 different long-chain branches amino acids. Each protein will have a unique combination of these amino acids and in turn, will provide different beneficial qualities. Contrary to a popular myth devised in the 60s, there aren't incomplete sources of protein in the foods we buy. For example, 100 grams of dark red kidney beans can contain 24-28 grams of protein, not 24-28 half grams. [9] Keeping that in mind, there are still eight essential amino acids that we need to consume, as we cannot produce them ourselves. These are the following:

- Isoleucine

- Leucine
- Lysine
- Methionine
- Phenylalanine
- Threonine
- Tryptophan
- Valine

Each one of these plays a different role in things like muscle repair or other bodily functions. There is no need to worry about obtaining adequate amounts of these unless you are a bodybuilder or have special circumstances. If you were eating a well-planned plant-based diet, it would be rarer for you to be lacking in one of these for a significant period. Each gram of protein comes out to about 4 calories. It takes a lot more energy for the body to digest protein. This is known as the **energy cost.** The energy cost of protein, however, is still not going to outweigh the energy it can provide. If you think eating only protein will burn calories, it will not. It will only cause metabolic distress, liver stress and damage, as well as other digestive issues.

Many of us are taught that in order for us to get enough protein we need to eat tons of meat and dairy because these are the best sources for them. This is factually inaccurate. Protein is actually found in many plant products that also come with an array of nutritionally beneficial qualities and minus all the saturated fat and cholesterol. According to WHO, processed meats are class 1 carcinogen that is in the same category as smoking. We will learn more about the dangers of saturated fat later on. In fact, if you really want to increase your insulin sensitivity while intermittent fasting a vegan diet is a great way to do so. (8) The American Diabetics Association has concluded that a vegan diet is appropriate and completely adequate to the stages in life namely: infancy, adolescence, pregnancy, and fetal development. (8) Vegan sources of protein can be found in a wide variety of foods that can make an endless combination of flavors and dishes; after all, there are over 39,000 different species of plants known globally. Check out the list to the below for some awesome plant-based sources of protein. Why consume products that nutritionally less efficient and at a higher cost to your wallet and more importantly, your health.

Food	Protein Content per 100g
Red Kidney Beans	28 grams
Green Lentils	9 grams
Quinoa	10-13 grams
Whole Wheat Pasta	15-25 grams
Nuts (almonds)	21 grams
Chia seeds	22 grams
Tofu	10 grams

So how much protein do you need on a daily basis? Well, that depends just like calories, on a wide variety of factors. You can calculate something called your Recommended Dietary Allowance (RDA), which can tell you how much protein you need at a **MINIMUM** in order for you not to get sick. This will also only calculate the RDA of a woman who is sedentary. The more physical activity, especially strength and/or endurance training, the more protein you will need. You can calculate your RDA with the following formula:

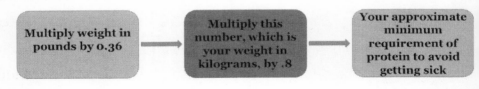

Remember not to use this as a daily recommendation but just to gain an idea of how much protein the female body does need to function.

Carbohydrates (Carbs)

Carbohydrates come in all shapes and forms but all of them are forms of sugars. They are a vital energy source for every human but too much of some and consuming large amounts at certain times of day can lead problems with weight, hormonal homeostasis, and other health issues. The types you should be aware of are **Monosaccharides, Disaccharides,** and **Non-starch/starch Polysaccharides** (dietary fiber). Each carbohydrate comes out to about 4 calories. However, in your daily life, you can just think about "simple carbs" and "complex carbs."

The starches and sugars are the sources of energy in food. These are the things that your body uses in the form of glucose, and glycogen when they are being directed to the liver, muscles and fat cells for storage. You could consider **Monosaccharides** as "good" sugar, ones that provide quality energy and that can be found in quality foods. Monosaccharides include glucose and fructose. These are found in things like vegetables, fruits, as well as in man-made glucose-fructose syrups. These all vary in sweetness depending on the individual monosaccharide and are

39

absorbed by the body without the need for extra digestive processes. Because organs like the brain or red blood cells cannot use fat and protein as energy, a baseline level of glucose must be present and for women, this approximately 130 grams per day. [10] Table sugar would be a **Disaccharide.** [10] Disaccharides, unlike monosaccharides that are directly absorbed by the small intestine, need to be broken down by digestive enzymes prior to entering the bloodstream as glucose. Then there are the **polysaccharides,** found in things like roots vegetables and grains. These too require further digestive processes in order for them to be used as energy but once converted they provide long-lasting and stable energy.

Whether you are fasting or not your diet should include a combination of both monosaccharides and polysaccharides in larger quantities than disaccharides. Simply put, eat more fruit and veggies just as your mama told you to. Fruits are amazing sources of monosaccharides and specifically fructose, you can taste them through the sweetness of the fruit, but polysaccharides typically are paired with more calorically dense ingredients like potatoes and yams. [11]

CARBOHYDRATES FAMILY	
Types of MONODOSACCHARIDES	
Fructose	Fruits, vegetables and honey
	Also derived from the digestion of sucrose
Glucose	Small amounts are found in some fruits, vegetables and honey
	Manufactured foods
	Digestion and conversion of other carbohydrates
Galactose	Digestion of Lactose
Types of DISACCHARIDES	
Sucrose	Derived from Sugar cane and sugar beet
	Sweet root vegetables such as beet root and carrots
	Table sugar, manufactured foods
Maltose	Malted wheat and barley
	Malt Extract
	Beer
Lactose	Milk
	Milk Products - Cheese, yogurt
Trehalose	Mushrooms and edible fungi
Types of POLYSACCHARIDES	
Starch	Cereal Foods
	Potato
	Small amounts in other root vegetables and unripe fruits
Non-Starch Polysaccharides	Vegetables and fruits
	Wholegrain cereals
	Pulses - Beans, lentils and etc

Now I know many of you have probably heard weird rules about what times of day when to and not to eat carbohydrates. Believe it or not, there may be some truth to these claims. Depending on what time of day and the type of activities you are doing that day carbohydrates can make a big difference. After a real work out session, for example, studies published in the *Journal of the International Society of Sports Nutrition* found that eating within 2 hours doubled the amount of glycogen storage occurring in the muscles. After the 2-hour mark, the amount of energy being stored away from your next meal is cut by 50%. [12] What can we take from these findings? Well, if your best interest is in reducing the amount of energy you consume that is stored then after a workout, it would be best to refrain from eating for an additional two hours. Of course, in this period, you will want to drink tons of water to keep somewhat full but mainly, to keep hydrated. Did you know women actually get hotter than their male counterparts do during exercise? This is probably due to the higher levels of blood volume women naturally have. [13]

During the premenstrual phase of your cycle, you will be experiencing a significantly higher level of both estrogen and progesterone. Do you remember those hormones? When they are at high levels they can lower total amount of blood in your body by 8%! Women who are on any form of chemical birth control can see significantly higher levels of estrogen and progesterone too. [13] You can increase your total blood level by staying drinking water throughout the entire day, especially in this phase of your cycle. Exercise is going to be a crucial factor in any weight loss journey as well as in any proper planning of an intermittent fasting regimen. We will get further into the knowledge needed in planning your unique intermittent fasting regimen in the next chapter. Exciting!

The subject of carbohydrates can be a lot to take in with everything we just covered but will still prove important informing a foundation of knowledge for you. On a daily basis, however, it is recommended to not stress about these details and simplify it. You can think of monosaccharides— things like fruits and veggies—as "simple sugars," and hardier foods like potatoes and whole grain pasta as "complex carbs." Both have their benefits, but timing will be key when choosing when to eat. Refer to the table above for how exercise and eating time are correlated when aiming for weight loss.

0-2 hours after exercise	The maximum amount of glycogen is kept in the muscles and then the liver and fat cells for use on another time.	Beneficial for weight gain and muscle recovery especially after vigorous exercises. Amino acid supplements containing zero sugars and calories can be taken in order to reduce muscle soreness without consuming excess glucose.
2 hours + after exercise	50% less glycogen stored	Beneficial for weight loss and allows your body to naturally redirect energy usage to previously stored glycogen in the liver, muscles, and fat.

Fats

Let us get some fat! Despite the bad rep fat has gotten over the years, it is an essential component in a healthy diet and plays crucial roles in bodily functions like your hormonal processes. As a woman, you carry around 6-11% more fat than your male counterparts do and your body is far more efficient at storing fat. This natural precautionary process, however, is in place to protect vital reproductive organs as well as possible fetal development, even if you are not pregnant. If we were still hunter-gatherers like all humans used to be, these thing would not be an issue. Yet in today's society, especially western society, the majority diet consists of calorie dense foods containing copious amounts of some **good** and mostly **bad fat**. A gram of fat contains approximately 9 calories. Multiply this by the 3-6 meals the average Westerner eats per day and you are getting dangerously high levels. Studies have shown in the fact that the average North American has fatty streaks in their arteries by the age of 10. Therefore, because your body has evolved to store this macronutrient, it can be a recipe for disaster.

On the other hand, women who become deficient in fat due to excess dieting, exercise, eating disorders or other circumstances can run into a whole lot of problems. A study was done at Harvard Cambridge found that body fat has a direct influence on female reproduction. Women who are underweight for longer periods of time can have drastic affect on the brain function. The part of your brain responsible for hormone production can become less efficient and damaged. This can lead you to have the same estrogen levels that a girl who hasn't gone through puberty yet. They also found that in girls and women who are way past or below a healthy weight for their age range can have a wide range of hormonal issues. These kinds of damages to the female reproductive system have the potential to be permanent as well as life-threatening in the future. This is why it is extremely important to keep a healthy balance of fat in your diet, and ideally only good fat.

Just as not all carbohydrates are the same, there are also different types of fats. There are four different types of fats in our diet: **saturated fats, monounsaturated fat, polyunsaturated fat,** and **trans fats.** It is important to know the difference between these because they all have significantly different aspects that will affect you as a woman.

Throughout this next section, you may see that I am strongly recommending a vegetarian or vegan diet for you. Without a doubt, eating these ways will eliminate some of the most harmful things you probably consume, but at the same time moderation is a great first step. You don't want to live a life where you feel trapped daily by your self-imposed rules. That's no way to live. On the other hand, new ways of eating will always take some effort to get used to and moderating your consumption of unhealthy products can be an amazing first step! For example, at first you could try something like going meat-free every second day or simply replacing your milk with almond milk. You can even buy both and mix them to slowly get used to the difference if you feel that will help you. Everyone is different and it is important to be self-aware and to have the goal of living your best life, because you only get one.

Saturated Fat: Bad Fat

This fat is found mostly in animal products, especially meat and dairy, with the exception of a few plant-based oils. It is generally solid at room temperature and it ends up solidifying after you absorb it. Saturated solidifies on the walls of your arteries restricting and eventually blocking blood flow which can cause a heart attack or stroke. Saturated fat plays no beneficial role in your health whatsoever. In fact, it harms you in numerous ways. The American Heart Association has now taken the stance that saturated fat and dietary cholesterol are both directly linked to heart disease, the #1 killer worldwide. In regards to obesity and diabetes, it has been clearly linked to increased insulin resistance while also raising LDL cholesterol levels, which also contribute to clogging arteries making it a key contributor. [16] Active research is also conducted right now on the links between saturated fat and Alzheimer's and Dementia. (17)

However, there is good news. You can reverse the changes this harmful substance has caused. By switching to a primary or completely plant-based diet, you are able to reverse the effects of heart disease to some degree. (18) This is mainly due to the complete elimination of bad cholesterol from the diet and the replacement of saturated fat with healthy unsaturated fats. Simply just reducing saturated fat intake showed minimal results compared to replacing them with plant-based sources. (16)

Monounsaturated and Polyunsaturated Fats

These are the fats that you're going to want to surround yourself with. Unsaturated fats are liquid at room temperature and sourced from plants, nuts, seeds, and some oils. When you consume adequate amounts of unsaturated fat and little to no saturated fat, you can improve cholesterol levels (reducing your LDL), ease inflammation, and **increase insulin sensitivity** as well as stabilizing heart rhythms. Both the American Heart Association and Harvard founded this information. (16)

Omega-3 fatty acids are a crucial type of **polyunsaturated** fat that you will want to include in your diet. When you hear "omega-3s", you probably think right away of fish as being an excellent source, you are not wrong [22]. However, this only refers to the amount per serving you can get. This is because every single fish not only contains mercury but they also come with a heaping portion of those devils saturated fat and cholesterol. Significant amounts of research are being done right now to see if it is even safe to eat fish after the Fukushima nuclear disaster in Japan in 2011. [23]

Omega-3 Fatty Acids and Women

These fats, however, come with a ton of benefits and especially when included in the diet of someone who is intermittently fasting. They even reduce the risks of breast cancer. (24) A cohort study with over 3,000 women showed that consumption of higher levels of omega-3 fatty acids, particularly EPA and DHA, "were to be associated with a 25% reduction in breast cancer reoccurrence." They have also shown high promise in numerous studies and one, in particular, was able to conclude that the regular utilization of these are actually effective when it comes to combatting menstrual pain than ibuprofen [25].

If you have been living your life constantly in a fed state and in turn have been storing glycogen on the regular, your liver is probably overworked and stuffed full of fat. When there is an excess of fat in the liver over long periods, you are at a very high risk of developing the non-alcoholic fatty liver disease (NAFLD). The regular consumption of these fats has shown to reduce not only the fat in your liver and thus reducing your risk but also reducing inflammation and any other infections.

Nevertheless, why are we hyping up omega-3 fatty acids so much in a book about intermittent fasting for women? This is because they actually have an effect on insulin resistance and sensitivity. Studies have shown it is an effective treatment (not cure) for individuals with metabolic syndrome. If you, however, have not developed issues like this or close to this, consuming these fats on a regular basis is a great and easy way to **support**

your insulin sensitivity. Combining this with an intermittent fasting regimen allows you to not only control insulin production by controlling energy consumption, but also by controlling what is in the energy that you actually do consume.

You can source these fatty acids from clean and humane sources such as flax seeds, walnuts, and other nuts as well as canola or soybean oil. You can also find plant-sourced supplements to take our omega-3s in pill form instead.

Trans Fats (Trans Fatty Acids)

While trans fats, or trans fatty acids, occur in a very small amount in nature, trans fats are in fact **industrially produced fats.** Trans fats are unique in that they are a "semi-solid" fat made by partially hydrating on a molecular level an unsaturated fat, typically this is done with vegetable oil. These partially hydrated oils (PHO), have been proven to cause dramatic increases in your LDL cholesterol (the bad one), and thus increase your risk for heart disease [34]. The discovery that hydrating fats was possible came in 1890, and by 1911, was already being widely used in the food industry. [34] This was because trans fats are actually a more stable version of unsaturated fats, which can become rancid when exposed to elements like heat, air, and light. Therefore, food manufacturers could expect much high-profit margins using the product. One product, in particular, was the main thing associated with trans fats for a long time and this was margarine. Margarine did not gain popularity due to lactose intolerance as you may think; it actually became popular in WWII due to the need to ration dairy butter. By 1980, products like lard were being replaced on a wide scale because people thought trans fats were actually healthier. [34] And girl they were wrong.

You know saturated fats are bad for you but in 1980 when clear links between saturated fat consumption and heart disease became prevalent, it drove a large growth in the utilization of trans fats as a replacement. [34] 10 years later, the evidence was clear that they brought an even greater risk of heart disease than saturated fats. Trans fats increase levels of your LDL cholesterol (dietary cholesterol) greater than saturated fats, increase the **accumulation of fat in blood vessels,** while also lower your HDL cholesterol. All of these consequences can lead not only to heart disease, but also to strokes, atherosclerosis, and diabetes (due to their damaging effect on the metabolic functions of the liver). [34]

Trans fats have a short dark history in human food consumption. Today, they are usually found in products like store made pastries, microwave popcorn, potato chips, and crackers. [24] Many places around the world have banned the sale of foods that contain PHOs. In Canada actually, partially hydrated oils are now prohibited nationwide [24]. Trans fats today are usually found in products like store made pastries, microwave popcorn, potato chips, and crackers. [24]

Types of Fat	Saturated Fat	Unsaturated Fat			
		Trans Fats	Monounsaturated Fats	Polyunsaturated Fats	
				Omega-3	Omega-6
Source	Animal fats and animal products (e.g: Whole milk, yogurt, red meat, butter, chocolate, tropical oils - coconut, palm	On the process of phasing out, but may still be available in processed, common in those with long shelf-life. Margarine, hydrogenated vegetable oil	Olive oil, sunflower oil, cashews, some beef fat, avacodos, oatmeal, popcorn, nut based oil	Found most in flax and hemp seed. Also found in soybean oil, sardines, salmon, mackerel, eggs, beans, broccoli, strawberriews	Poultry, nuts, cereals, durum wheat, whole grains, vegetable oil (Corn, soybean, sunflower oil)
Should you eat?	Raise both LDL and HDL. Increase total cholesterol. May increase risk of heart disease. Eat no more than 16-20 grams of saturated fat a day/ 2000 calorie diet	Avoid like the plague! Raise LDL (bad cholesterol) and lower HDL (good cholesterol). Increase risk of heart disease, stroke and diabetes	Recommended over saturated fats. Lower LDL and raise HDL. Lower risk of heart disease. Source of vitamin E	High Omega 3 to 6 ratio is optimum for reducing heart disease and anti inflamation	

Vitamins/Minerals

Vitamins and mineral play a crucial role in anyone's healthy diet. As a woman there a few that you will want to take extra steps to make sure you are getting adequate amounts. This is the case for things like Iron. Especially women with heavier periods are at higher risks of iron deficiency. You can make sure you are getting iron by eating many leafy greens, the darker the green the better, and cooking your food in iron cast skillets!

While vitamins play a huge role in our diet, nowadays it is more than easy to make sure you are getting enough of them. A multivitamin supplement will be something you want in all methods of intermittent fasting. You will see later on in the sample weekly nutritional tracker that a multivitamin column is included. This is to stress the need for regular vitamin consumption during **any** fasting regimen.

What to Avoid

We have already lightly touched on a few things you should avoid but it has been spread out and we need to get more into depth. Because you will probably be consuming a limited number of calories while intermittent fasting, you should try to make every calorie that you do consume to be beneficial. Of course, it's still possible to consume excess calories while practicing IF, but generally if portion sizes are kept the same, you will enter a calorie deficit. This can be done by eliminating harmful nutrients and food sources from your diet. The importance of staying away from saturated fat and dietary cholesterol needs to be stressed. Not only will these not benefit goals of both weight loss or gaining lean mass but they will also increase your risk for heart attack, congestive heart defect, stroke, obesity, diabetes, possibly Alzheimer's and Dementia. The easiest way to do this is by eliminating animal products from your diet. Saturated fat is found only in meat and dairy products and dietary cholesterol is even more exclusive to this group.

In fact, as a woman practicing intermittent fasting, you will most likely want to stay away from dairy products especially. All dairy products contain hormones because they come from a live pregnant animal, and these hormones have the potential to disrupt endocrine processes and thus have massive impacts on your entire body. These hormones include progesterone, estrogen, and steroids, which are showing possible links to cancers. [25] In dairy products, milk contains the lowest concentration of these hormones, followed by yogurt, then cheese and butter. Some of the alternatives to cow's milk are soymilk and almond milk. You can also create a nut milk at home easily too.

If your goal is to shed some pounds, then you will need to have a diet higher in **unsaturated** fats and protein with lower levels of carbohydrates. In doing so, you are restricting the addition of extra energy into your body. During a fast, your body will be depending on the previously made fat-stores as its primary energy source. Consuming more protein and fat will, in turn, support the body's ability to use fat as an energy source. To be clear, you will want higher amounts of **unsaturated fats.**

You will also want to avoid the conventional snack foods that are notorious glucose pumpers. Things like chocolate have copious amounts of sugar that are going to cause you to have massive glucose spikes followed by crashes. Things like potato chips are typically extremely high in salt which dehydrates you significantly, the contrary of what you want to happen while intermittent fasting. The following list contains several common sources of the things you want to avoid and an easy replacement for them.

Foods to Avoid	Reasons	Easy Replacements
Meat	Contains high levels of saturated fat and cholesterol and is classified as a class 1 carcinogen by the World Health Organization.	Tofu, beans, jackfruit, lentils, quinoa, chickpeas, soy, and faux meat products. Soy and faux meat products are typically extremely high in protein in order to combat the common misbelief that plants do not contain protein.
Dairy Products	Have a high potential of disrupting your brain function and hormones due to the hormonal content inside the products. They also typically contain high levels of saturated fat and cholesterol.	Soymilk, oat milk, almond milk, rice milk, cashew milk, plant-based cheeses, and yogurts. Avocado also makes a great substitute to create creamy textures in foods.
Eggs	There is a lot of controversy around eggs still in the scientific literature. However, we still know eggs have extremely high amounts of dietary cholesterol that is directly linked to heart disease according to the AHA.	Plant-based egg substitutes are available in some locations. As for cooking, however, there are tons of great egg replacements with very workable flavors. Some of these include bananas, avocado, applesauce, and arrowroot powder.
Processed Sugar	Processed sugar is everything you want to avoid while intermittent fasting. Processed sugar will provide you with the exact large doses of glucose that you attempt to avoid.	Beets, dates, and fruits.

How to Track Your Nutritional Values

Tracking your nutrition does not have to be a massive task. On a daily basis, it can be as complex as you are comfortable with. We went over earlier how many calories you as a woman would need and it really depends on your lifestyle.

To track your nutrients accurately, I really recommend getting a digital kitchen scale to weigh your food, even if you only want to track your calories. This is because in most cases a beneficial and healthful diet will include plentiful ingredients that do not come with nutrition labels. However, we do have apps for that, apps and Google. Many apps will have a large database that contains huge varieties of foods and their nutritional values, some also even let scan the barcode of certain products in stores so they can be extremely helpful.

There are tons of apps out there for you to use but I really recommend checking out "chronometer." Chronometer has an advanced database that has a ridiculous amount of nutritional values even between different brands and serving methods. Of course a kitchen scale will still be a very handy tool, but a chronometer can do all the math and tracking for you.

One app I have used in the past even calculated my micronutrients and showed me them in levels of percentages so everything was so easy to track. This also helps with motivation because for many of us there is a need to "fill things up" to 100%. In addition, simply searching "calories in an apple" can give you the ability to calculate how many calories are for the apple you are eating. Therefore, if you do not have an app, you can just prepare your portion size of any given ingredient, weigh the ingredient and then google how many calories are in 100 grams of [put ingredient here]. Then you can write it down in a notebook that is easy to take everywhere or even just the notes app on your phone on a daily basis. Then at the end of every week, it will be helpful to add up all your macronutrients and calories for the week, along with your progress on your regimen. The following table is a great way for you to track everything important neatly so you can reference them later and see your progress.

Weekly Tracker							
Week	Calories	Protein (g)	Carbs (g)	Fats (g)	Multi-Vitamin?	Goals Met?	Notes
1					Yes/No	Yes/No	
2					Yes/No	Yes/No	
3					Yes/No	Yes/No	
4					Yes/No	Yes/No	
5					Yes/No	Yes/No	

The first steps you will want to take when **you decide to start tracking your nutrition** is measuring all of your **current levels** and then formulating your **desired levels and base levels**. By "levels" I do not mean weight, body fat %, or anything like that. I mean the numerical levels of your nutrition.

58

For example, if I am eating 2200 calories every day, my current calorie level would be 2200. When you calculate a level you will want to include your calories, protein, fat, and carbs. Your current levels will allow you to see EXACTLY where you are now and from there you can make educated decisions on how to proceed. The current levels should include a wide range of different components in your life. To do this accurately, I recommend changing nothing about your life for a week and just tracking it all. You should track the foods you eat, the calories that come with them, the times of day you eat or feel hungry, the amount of exercise you are doing in a day, and the times you wake up and go to sleep. Also, keep aware of the places and types of food you are eating. This is a great way to gain some self-awareness on your habits and of your weaknesses. We will get more into self-awareness later on.

Once you have gone through a week of tracking your current levels, you now will have the information you need to formulate your **base levels**. Your base levels refer to the minimum amount of macronutrients, and more importantly calories, that you need in order for you not to get sick. This part will be an **extremely vital** part of any successful practicing faster. Because you will be eating very infrequently, you have to know the minimum amount of nutrients you need to obtain in order for all bodily and hormonal functions to keep working properly. The chart in *Chapter 4: Nutrition and Intermittent Fasting* that shows calorie intake based on age, is a reference to check once you calculate your own unique base levels. If your calculated level deviates extremely from those levels it might be a good idea to re-calculate. On the other hand, some women will have significantly different baselines based on their lifestyle. I recommend that once you calculate your base levels, you increase them by 2-5% so that you can be confident you will reach adequate nutrition. Aim for the moon and land with the stars.

Your **desired levels** depend completely on you as an individual. Do you want to lose weight at a certain rate? Then how close do you want to be to your **base levels** on a daily basis? On the other hand, if you are trying to gain weight or muscle mass, how far away do you want to be from your **base levels?** For reference, a woman who is trying to lose 1 pound per week would have to burn 3,500 calories in that week or consume a lesser amount of calories, or somewhere in-between.

Staying Hydrated

Before we move on from nutrition, we need to cover the important role water will play in any method of fasting you choose. practice and there are heavy concentrations of A lot of people in the Middle East and Africa, some of the hottest places on Earth. How do these people not survive but thrive while fasting in the desert? One benefiting factor is staying completely hydrated. [33]

Staying hydrated allows you to maintain healthy blood levels and pressure levels while also improving brain function, organ function, and has numerous cosmetic benefits as well. In fact, after significant time spent intermittent fasting with a healthy primarily plant-based diet, you can expect clearer complexion and smoother skin. This is especially true when hydrated. Daily, even if you are not exercising, you should aim for 8-10 glasses of water per day.

Meal Preps Make Everything Easier

Many methods of intermittent fasting include a significant portion of the day fasted (you are actually fasting as you sleep every night). Because of this, however, you will not want to have to cook your meal packed with quality and clean ingredients, and then clean the dishes and all that nonsense that comes with the whole ordeal. Instead, you can concentrate all of this dirty work into between 2-5 hours per week, total. If you really think about it, we spend huge portions of our day thinking about what and when we are going to eat, prepping or traveling to get there, and cleaning afterward or spending extra money (which is just time produced energy). The combination of fasting and meal prepping can literally give you several hours extra per week.

To meal prep successfully, you will need to know the above-mentioned levels in Chapter 4. Once you know all that you need to know about your own macronutrients and caloric intake, it's time to think of what foods you like to eat that fit into those parameters. Remember that no matter what, unless you happen to be unfortunately allergic, you will want tons of fruits and veggies. Now you can form your meal plan for the week based on the method of fasting you choose to practice. We will go over the most common methods in the following chapter.

The first step in any meal prep is to divide your meal plan is to divide your preps into 2-3 cooking sessions per week. You should not prep your food for more than **4** days in advance for more reasons than it is gross to eat stale stuff. Cooked food actually loses its nutritional content over time. The longer your tomato pasta sauce sits in the fridge the more and more nutrients it will lose. Specifically, the more micronutrients will be lost. Calories, protein, and carbohydrates are relatively stable nutrients and it would take significant decomposition to affect these. Fat, on the other hand, is also relatively stable but possess the possibility of turning rancid. But for the ones that are lost, these nutrients aren't actually "disappearing" or even just evaporating, but they can be sensitive to air, temperature, and even light. (26) Research at Penn State showed that fresh spinach lost around 53% of its folate content after 8 days that was at 39 degrees Fahrenheit too. Try not to get overwhelmed with knowing what things like "folate" are. This is just an example to show how food can lose nutritional value over time in storage. They concluded that cooling does lower that rate of loss in many foods but the loss is still inevitable. Some of their findings for specific nutrients can be found in the table below:

Nutrients	Sensitivities
Proteins and Carbohydrates	Relatively stable macronutrients
Fats	Air, light, and heat
Vitamin A	Air, light, and heat
Vitamin C	Air, light, and heat (this vitamin is particularly unstable)
Vitamin B-6	Light and heat
Folic Acid	Air, light, and heat (this vitamin is particularly unstable)
Thiamin	Air and heat
Riboflavin	Light and heat [26]

Therefore, to prevent you from wasting food or eating nutritionally inadequate food, you should not prep your food for more than 4 days in advance. Choose how many cooking sessions you will have per week. I like Sunday preps for Monday to Thursday and Thursday preps from Fridays to Sundays. That is 4-day prep, followed by 3-day prep. Many people will also limit their prep to 6 days a week and allow themselves to eat out for one meal a week, which can be up to you.

While you are actually prepping your food, it will be helpful to follow this order of steps. This will allow you to be as efficient as possible.

Reading Nutrition Labels

This is basic but there are myths and confusions out there that are important to address. When you look at a label, you will most likely see something that says 'Daily Value.' This is a term to describe what the 'average' person needs and should really be **ignored.** The average person is based on minimal data from a wide population and doesn't necessarily take individual factors into account. These levels are really only calculated on averages and contain a lot of assumptions. For example, a granola bar may say it gives you 25% of your Vitamin C, but 25% one woman's daily value will probably be very different from another man's daily value.

The **FIRST** thing you want to look at on a nutrition label is the saturated fat and cholesterol content. The fat on most nutritional labels will typically list "Fat" as unsaturated fat and "+Sat. Fat" is typically directly beneath. Get in the habit of putting anything with either of these back on the grocery shelf.If the label passes the first test, for the **SECOND,** check the portion size and calories per portion. **THIRD,** look at the calories, carbs, proteins, and good fat content. The grams of protein listed on these nutrition labels are "complete grams" of protein and do not ever only contain "partial proteins" because there is no such thing. **Finally,** scan the vitamins and minerals, and the ingredients section for anything that is potentially harmful.

On To The Meal Prep

Now it's time to start talking about the meal prep itself – we have already dealt with macronutrients and food types: now it's time to start putting it all together.

What Kinds Of Foods Can Be Cooked Together

This is where a lot of newbie meal preppers get stuck - they don't take into account that different types of foods require different cooking times. The result is that some parts of the meal are overdone, while other parts taste raw.

When doing meal prep, it is important to realize that some foods take longer to cook than others. Carrots, for example, take longer to cook than spinach. Different cuts of meat also require different handling – for example, chuck steak or brisket takes longer to cook than rump steak because it has more connective tissue that needs to be broken down.

So, if you were to make a meal using brisket, for example, and you wanted to add broccoli, you would have to wait until the meat was halfway cooked before you could add the broccoli, or it would become a mushy mess.

If, on the other hand, you had a tougher vegetable, like a carrot, you could add it earlier in the cooking time. A good rule of thumb to follow is that the tougher and denser the vegetable or meat is, the longer the cooking time.

Meal Prep Instructions (General)

Step 1: Preheat your oven to your needed temperature and start to bring any liquids to a boil that you may need.

Step 2: Weigh out all your ingredients and track them in your respective journal.

Step 3: Organize your ingredients from the longest cook time to shortest cook times. Typically, you should start with the carbohydrates of each meal, with some exceptions.

Pro tip: While planning your meal, try to choose common base ingredients that can be used for more than one meal. For example, on four-day meal prep, while you are fasting, you could prepare enough rice for 2-3 meals all at once and still have room in your other meals for variety in your diet.

Step 4: Lay out all Tupperware or food containers that you will need.

Step 5: Bake and boil ingredients that are cooked this way as they typically take the longest i.e. potatoes and yams

Step 6: While these ingredients cook, start the ingredients that take less time to cook. Typically, things that are fried or gradually heated on stovetop i.e. beans.

Step 7: As each ingredient finishes cooking, place it in their corresponding container but let it cool before covering it. Placing the lead on the container can further cook your food, removing further nutrients, and when cooled in your fridge can cause it to become soggy. Who wants to eat a wet and soggy stir-fry?

Step 8: Clean and pack away all your food. You have just prepped 4 days' worth of food and now will only have one or two containers that need to be washed on a daily basis.

It is best to make a bullet form list or a small table to lay out your meals and meal times for the week. Making a bullet form list as you think of meals can be a great way to organize your thoughts and see the variety of foods in your week, and putting this data into a table can help you organize the times when you eat these foods. On the next page, you can refer to the examples when you yourself are in the planning stage.

Safety First

Now, you might be wondering why you needed to write the date on the meals before they were frozen. The reason is safety. Freezing enables us to extend the shelf-life of cooked foods. Even frozen, though, they will not last forever.

Here is a guide to the shelf-life of your frozen cooked meals:

1. **Casseroles and stews**: 2-3 months
2. **Soups, stocks, and broths**: 2-3 months
3. **Fish**: 3 months
4. **Meat or poultry**: 2-6 months
5. **Gravy**: 2-3 months
6. **Pizza**: 1-2 months
7. **Pasta**: 2 months

When in doubt, err on the side of caution. If you are not sure how long a food has been in the freezer, it is safer to throw it out. If food is freezer-burned, it won't taste good when eaten, so throw it out.

A good rule of thumb is to make sure that nothing stays in your freezer longer than 2-3 months. Put the date bought/made on everything that you freeze and check your freezer regularly so that you use older items first.

Also, when packing your freezer, take some time to haul everything out – I know it is a pain – and repack so that the new items are at the bottom or in the back and the older items are the first ones you reach for.

Tools To Consider

You do not need every gadget on the market. What you should do before going out to buy the latest of everything is think about whether or not you are going to use it.

Take a spiralizer, for example. It is quite nice to have if you like zoodles or to slice beetroot finely for a salad. Is it essential, though? Beware of the "trendy" items; there is no point getting them if you don't plan on using them.

Essential Tools

These will depend on the types of food you are going to make, but the following are fairly standard:

1. **Large pots and pans**: To reduce your workload overall, it makes sense to double up every recipe you make. You are going to need bigger pots and pans to make this possible. At the very least, you need to get one large skillet and a stock pot.

2. **Lots of freezer-safe containers/resealable bags**: You're cooking large quantities of food; you will need to be able to refrigerate/freeze it until needed.

3. **A permanent marker and labels**: This might not sound like something you need in the kitchen, but you'll see its value when you have a freezer full of food that you cannot identify. Make a label for each container/bag with the name of the meal and the date it was made.

4. **A slow cooker**: This is a tool that is not strictly essential, but that will make your life a whole lot easier, especially if you are short on time. What is nice about the slow cooker is that you can literally set it and forget it. It

is difficult to burn your food in one and even the toughest cuts of meat will come out butter soft. What can be a pain is that it takes hours to cook anything. So, you could prep meals for the slow cooker ahead of time and freeze them. You'd need to take them out the evening before you want to make them so that they can thaw properly. Then it's simply a case of putting them into the slow cooker, setting it on low, and by the time you get home from work, the food will be cooked.

5. **An instant pot**: This again is not strictly necessary, but it can be useful for the meal prepper because it allows you to make large meals in a much shorter time frame.

6. **A food processor**: When you are preparing a small meal for your family, a food processor may seem like a luxury. When it comes to hour three of chopping vegetables during a meal prep session, however, you'll understand why this is an essential tool.

7. **A great set of knives**: You want to spend a little money here and get a great set of knives. This will make not only topping and tailing veggies easier, but also allow you to joint chickens, etc. Great knives help to make meal prep a breeze.

8. **A good kitchen scale and set of measuring cups/jugs**: You need accurate equipment to make sure that the recipes are made properly.

As you can see, there are not a lot of items on the essential tool list. For your own meal prep journey, pick those that make the most sense to you.

Example Meal Plan List (Crescendo Method)

Monday (Feeding Day)

- Applesauce, granola, blueberries
- Yams and chickpeas
- Pasta and tomatoes

Tuesday (Fasting Day)

- Bananas, hummus, and pita

Wednesday (Feeding Day)

- Tofu scramble with veggies
- Tomato soup and a spinach sandwich
- Kidney bean stew with veggies

Thursday (Fasting day)

- Fruit smoothie and chopped veggies (carrots broccoli, celery)

Friday (Feeding Day)

- Applesauce, granola, mangos, and kiwi
- Lentil curry on rice

Saturday (Fasting day)

- Pineapples, strawberries, and peanut butter toast

Sunday (Feeding Day)

- Applesauce, granola, blueberries,
- Tofu stir-fry
- **REWARD MEAL (anywhere or anything you please)**

Chapter 5: Common Intermittent Fasting Variations

Now that you know what intermittent fasting is and benefits it can provide, maybe it is time to try it. As a starting point, it is good to look at a few of these several common methods and variations of IF, then if need be applying it to your unique circumstances. The schedules and lifestyles of a stay at home mom, a doctor, and a bartender would all have very different schedules and thus may have to choose different methods.

When looking through the methods it is important to keep in mind your daily life and schedule. As you read each way of fasting, try and picture yourself doing this and honestly tell yourself if you think this method is not only your favorite but also sustainable. You may love the look of one method, but it may conflict with other aspects of your life and you will need to adjust for that.

The 16:8 Method

This method involves you restricting food consumption within an eight-hour period and fasting what remained of the time/hours every day. This method is not a bad method at all to start with if you are a beginner. The 8-hour window allows for a lot of flexibility and that can mean less of a drastic change to your life as it is now. This method still gives you the benefits of fasting because your insulin levels are able to drop and stabilize for two-thirds of the day. In the other third portion of the day, much of the energy you consume will be used right away and not stored for later. It is always convenient to include your sleep time in your fasting window and it is actually recommended. When you sleep, you already have higher levels of Human Growth Hormone and fasting increases your secretion of it as well. (27) (28) Human Growth Hormone can promote cellular regeneration and more importantly for you, can promote healthy weight loss. (28) (29)

Ways to Implement the 16:8 Fasting Method		
Eating Time per Day: 8 Hours	**Fasting Time per Day: 16 Hours**	**Benefits**
Eat between 11 AM and 7 PM	Fast between 7 PM and 11 AM	If you go to sleep at around 10PM and wake up between 6-7AM, a majority of your fasting time will be while you are asleep. This particular method is nice if you lack an appetite in the morning and are generally hungrier at conventional lunch and dinner times.
Eat between 7 AM and 3 PM	Fast between 3 PM and 7 AM	If you are typically hungrier in the mornings or the middle of your day requires physical activity, then this method can allow you to eat when you wake up and burn the calories you ate in this period for the rest of the day. This may take more willpower and determination because a significant portion of you awake time will be spent fasted.
Eat between 3 PM and 11 PM	Fast between 11 PM and 3 PM	For some, this method may work, however, keep in mind that if you are consuming energy right before you go to sleep you will in turn store that energy and possibly slow or hinder your weight loss process.

The 24 Hour Fast & the 5:2 Diet

Then there is the 24-hour fasting method. This involves you fasting in a twenty-four-hour period one to two times per week. This would restrict your weekly total caloric intake, however, will do little to increase your insulin sensitivity and act as a sustainable form of bad weight gain prevention. For the 5 days that you are eating food in this method, you will be eating the standard diet and constantly be in a fed state. While the total caloric deficit may result in weight loss when also paired with exercise, this may be a damaging and irresponsible method of fasting and better referred to as controlled starving. Because as you now know from Chapter 3, any stage past **Phase II** in the **transition between the fed state and fasted state**, it can start to diminish cell function and hormonal processes. Any method that requires you as a woman to fast for a period longer than 24-hours in most cases will cause hormonal dysfunction and you could run into a series of problems due to this as mentioned before.

Ways to Implement the 24-hour Fasting Method		
Eating	**Fasting**	**Benefits**
Eat regularly from Thursday to Saturday and Monday and Tuesday.	Fast on Sunday and Wednesday.	You will most likely experience a caloric deficit and thus weight loss over time but this method does more closely represent controlled starvation or a crash diet. You also have less of an effect on increasing insulin sensitivity.

The 5:2 method or protocol is very similar to the 24-hour fast with the exception of an 8-hour eating window on fasting days while also restricting calories on these days to approximately 500 calories.

Ways to Implement the 5:2 Fasting Method		
Eating	**Fasting**	**Benefits**
Eat regularly from Thursday to Saturday and Monday and Tuesday. On fasting days, restrict calories to approximately 500 calories.	Fast between 10 AM and 6 PM on Sundays and Wednesdays.	While this is safe than the 24-hour fasting method, you still hinder your influence on insulin sensitivity compared to other methods.

Alternate Day Fasting method

The alternate day fasting method is another flexible plan confirmed as a safe weight loss method in both obese and simply overweight adults. (30) In this method, you can eat regularly every other day and practice a complete fast or restrict the other days to approximately 500 calories. The eating to fasting ratio throughout the week in this method will allow for a significant influence on your insulin production. However, like some ways of practicing, the alternate day fasting method can take more willpower as you will be spending an extensive amount of time awake and fasting. This may be especially difficult at first.

Ways to Implement the Alternate Day Fasting		
Eating	**Fasting**	**Benefits**
Eat regularly every other day.	Fast or consume a maximum of 500 calories on every other day.	This is a great method to try with very simple parameters as long as you have enough willpower and determination to resist cheating on fasted days.

The Warrior Diet

The Warrior diet is an interesting variation where you consistently limit yourself to one meal per day. This diet was created by an ex Israeli Special Forces named Ori Hofmekler in 2001. He has stated that it is based on the diet ancient warriors used to have, eating little to no food in the days and indulging with feasts at night. In modern times, the diet has been crafted to formal parameters of 20 hours spent fasting and 4 hours spent feeding but the feeding is intended to happen in the later portion of the day.

Ways to Implement Warrior Diet Fasting Method		
Eating	**Fasting**	**Benefits**
Eat for a 4-hour window on a daily basis in the later portion of the day. This meal will consist of a minimum of 2,000 calories for most individuals.	Fast or consume a maximum of 500 calories on for the other 12 hours you are awake. If your sleeping schedule does not allow for 8 hours, make sure you adjust so you can fast for 20 hours total.	This is widely accepted as the safest method for women new to intermittent fasting. The Crescendo method will ease your body and hormonal processes into the new trends you are creating in regards to insulin production.

While all of the above methods are common methods of intermittent fasting, as a woman I strongly encourage you to start with the Crescendo fasting method. Not only will it be an easier transition on your mind and body while still having beneficial effects on insulin sensitivity but it will also work well with many typical schedules. For instance, if you work the average 9-5 job, with this method you could consume food in the morning for breakfast, and lunch or an early dinner.

Crescendo Fasting Method (#1 RECOMMENDED METHOD FOR ANY WOMAN)

You may remember we mentioned this at the beginning of the book, the crescendo fasting method. With some very basic research, it is easy to see that this is one of the most widely recommended intermittent fasting methods for women. This is a fact for a number of reasons. The crescendo fasting method allows you to ease yourself into the **art of intermittent fasting** while still providing you with significant periods of fasting that will have the benefits on your insulin sensitivity. Because you as a woman have to take extra precautions when fasting due to the effects it can have on your hormones, the crescendo fasting method has been #1 recommended method for women to safely transition into this lifestyle change. Similar to the abovementioned '16:8' method, this method might be even better for you. With this method, you eat in 8-12 hour windows 4 days a week and fast for 12-16 hour windows 3 days per week.

Ways to Implement Crescendo Fasting Method		
Eating	**Fasting**	**Benefits**
Eat for 8-hour windows on Monday, Wednesday, Friday, and Sunday.	Fast or consume a maximum of 500 calories on Tuesday, Thursday and Saturday.	This is widely accepted as the safest method for women who are new to intermittent fasting. The Crescendo method will ease your body and hormonal processes into the new trends you are creating in regards to insulin production.

Rules for Crescendo Fasting

1. Fast only 2 or 3 days a week on non-consecutive days. For instance, fast on Tuesdays, Fridays, and Sundays.
2. Fast for 12 to 16 hours only. Do not exceed 16 hours if you can help it.
3. On your fasting days try and do some workouts such as yoga or walking.
4. On other days, do heavier workouts such as cardio or weight training.
5. You are allowed to take lots of water, tea, and coffee as long as they are free of added sugar, sweeteners, or milk.
6. Consider taking 5 – 8 grams of BCAA (branch chain amino acids) on your fast days. They contain very little calories yet provide much-needed fuel to your muscles.

These amino acids also take the edge off hunger and fatigue.

Chapter 6: Starting Your Intermittent Fast

Now that you have spent some time going through this guidebook and learning more about intermittent fasting, the next challenge is going to begin. It is time to actually start your intermittent fast. Many people are curious as to what they should affect when they get started with fasting, and they may have a lot of questions along the way. This chapter is going to take some time to discuss intermittent fasting and what followers should come to expect when they start on this eating method.

What can you expect?

Many people wonder what they should expect when they get started with fasting. They have spent most of their lives hearing that fasting is bad for them and that they shouldn't even consider that kind of eating plan. While most of the negatives about fasting are incorrect, it is still a good idea to know what will happen during your first few weeks on this kind of eating plan.

During the first few days, you may not notice much of a difference. The hunger may be a bit harder to deal with because your bod wants the constant stream of glucose that we talked about before. But because of your motivation and excitement about the fast and its results, you will probably feel pretty normal when it comes to those first few days and getting started with the fast.

After those first few days, things may get a bit more difficult. The body doesn't like that you have taken away that easy source of glucose. It likes having glucose present all the time because that glucose is an easy source of energy that you can burn through, even if it isn't that efficient and often gets stored in the body. In response, you may notice that you have a lot of cravings, you are really hungry (even abnormally so), and you will get headaches, stomach aches, and more.

Day three to five are often considered the more difficult when it comes to an intermittent fast. These are the days when the body starts to catch on to what you are doing, and it doesn't like it. It doesn't want to switch over to burning up fat, or it may even take some time before the body starts to burn through anything else. As the body runs out of carbs to consume, you will experience mood swings, irritability, headaches, low blood sugars, hunger, and lots of intense cravings. You may also be really tired and worn out because the body doesn't know where to turn to get the fuel it needs.

Most people are only going to deal with these side effects for a few days at most. The body will adapt pretty quickly and then you will be able to get over these side effects and feel better than before. Others may need to adjust for a little longer. It is a good idea to plan on spending the majority of the first week or so feeling a little rough and taking it easy.

The good news is that if you are able to get through this part of the intermittent fast, then this is the hardest part. Your body is going to adjust to not having that constant source of glucose available and you will start to see results. Within a week or so, your energy levels will go up, and when you step on the scale, you will start to notice that you have lost a lot of weight. That week can be tough, and there are a lot of people who end up quitting the fast because that part was so hard for them.

After that first week, you will find that staying on an intermittent fast can be pretty simple. You may want to consider working on a meal plan to go with the fast to ensure that you are eating the right number of calories and getting plenty of nutrition, both on your fasting days and on your regular eating days. But by this time, the fast should become a part of your regular lifestyle and you can follow it without noticing that much anyway.

After a while on the fast, you may want to take some time to evaluate your fast and see how it is working for you. If you find that it is still working well for you, that it fits into your lifestyle well, and you are still seeing weight and fat loss, then just stick with it and keeping using that method. But if you find that your weight loss is stalling, then you may want to consider upping the fast, even just temporarily, and seeing if that can help. So, if you are on the 16/8 fast, consider switching to a lower eating window, such as 20/4, or go to the eat, stop, eat plan. Even doing that for a week or so can turn the metabolism up some more and can give you more of the results that you want.

For most people, the fast will not be that difficult to follow, once they get through that initial stage where they need to let the body adapt. Once you get through some of those side effects, which usually lasts less than a week, you are going to be so amazed by the great benefits that come from the fast. You can always change up some of the methods that you use to ensure that you see some amazing results, even after the body has gotten used to the fasting method you choose to use.

What body and mental cues should you listen to?

This guidebook has spent some time talking about intermittent fasting and some of the benefits that come with it. Many people are able to go on an intermittent fast and after a few days at most, they will see a lot of improvements in their weight, their health, and so much more. But for others, an intermittent fast isn't going to be the best idea for them. Their body may not be able to adjust all that well or they may run into other issues. Some signs that you may need to get off your intermittent fast, especially if they keep showing up three to four weeks into the fast, include:

- When you always feel tired: Your body should adjust to the fast pretty quickly. You may feel tired for the first few days, but then the body will start to adjust and feel better. In fact, many people who go on this kind of eating plan experience a surge in energy after their body gets used to it. If you continue to feel tired and can't seem to get out of bed most days, then it may be time to readjust the eating plan or consider a different diet plan for you.

- When you are cranky for no reason or irritable: A little bit of irritability in the beginning is pretty normal. Your body wants to get that constant source of glucose back to itself, but you are taking it away, at least for a little bit. If you go on the ketogenic diet as well, you will find that you are really reducing the amount of glucose all the time. the body will be tired and won't know how to deal with this. But if your hormones are having a hard time regulating and you can't seem to deal with the mood swings and more, then it may be time to consider whether the fast is right for you or not.

- When your time of the month stops: In women, it is important to make sure to watch your cycle. If it starts to become really irregular or it stops altogether, then it is time to get off the intermittent fast right away.

- When you can't seem to concentrate or keep getting headaches: Many people respond to fasting with clearer mental focus and concentration. But some people find that the lack of glucose can give them big sugar crashes and headaches that just won't go away. If you can't get the headaches to go away after a few weeks of adjusting to the lack of constant glucose supply, then it may be a good idea to either change up the fast, or consider trying out a different type of diet plan.

- When constipation becomes an issue: A little bit of constipation in the beginning can be normal and is just a sign that you need to get some more fiber, and maybe other nutrients, into your body. But if you still deal with issues with your bowels and with other stomach issues, then it may be time to look into stopping an intermittent fast. Intermittent fasting can be so wonderful for so many people, but you may have some digestive issues to deal with when constipation becomes a bigger problem.

For most people, intermittent fasting is a great way to lose weight and improve their health. But for some people, fasting is not the best option. They may feel sick, deal with constipation, or have issues with other parts of their body. If any of the side effects above do happen to you (which is rare) or you feel off in another way, it may be time to reconsider whether intermittent fasting is the right option for you.

What are common mistakes to avoid?

There are a lot of great benefits that come with your intermittent fast. It can help you to lose a lot of weight without a lot of work. It can help to improve the health of your heart. It can even help with how well your brain functions, getting rid of diabetes, and so much more. With that said, there are a few mistakes that followers may do, sometimes without thinking, that can really ruin the results that you can see while fasting. Some of the most common mistakes that are made while fasting include:

- You continue to eat a lot of junk foods: While it is fine to have a little treat on occasion when fasting, if you continue to keep your diet primarily full of junk and processed foods, then you won't see any of the benefits of the fast. You need to make sure that your diet that is full of healthy nutrients to fill you up and help support the body when it is losing weight. Stick with healthy product, lots of healthy protein, whole grains (unless you follow a ketogenic diet), and good sources of dairy.

- You don't keep yourself busy: If you sit around all day watching the clock, getting through an intermittent fast is going to seem impossible. Idle hands are your worst enemy during this time. make sure that when you are on

89

a fast, you schedule something where you won't be around, or even think about food, this helps to keep the temptations, and even the hunger at bay.

- You abuse stimulants: Many intermittent fasters end up drinking coffee instead of breakfast. The usual recommendation is to have a cup or two in the morning because it can fight off hunger and help increase metabolism of fat. While having a few cups is just fine, you do not need to go crazy and get hooked onto coffee. Consider cutting it off by noon through so you don't get too dependent on it and you can let the caffeine subside long before bedtime.

- You are ambitious to start: It is good to be ambitious and excited about going on an intermittent fast. But if you jump on board too quickly, and take on something that is too much, it can be hard to maintain. Many people want to see the benefits right away. So they jump on with alternate day fasting or one of the Warrior diets and find that it is too hard to maintain. Building up with one of the easier versions, such as the 5:2 diet or 16/8 method, can make it much easier to get going with intermittent fasting and stick with it.

- You think that more has to be better: Some people think that intermittent fasting is great, so why not extend out the fast to two or three days? The issue with this is that most of the benefits that come with fasting will diminish after you go over 20 hours. Intermittent fasting relies on not going much more than 24 hours. This ensures that you get all of the benefits of fasting, without taking it too far and making it so you start to deal with starvation mode and other issues.

How do you maintain this Lifestyle?

Following an intermittent fast is not meant to be difficult. This is a process that you can easily utilize in any lifestyle that you have. Maintaining it is the best way to receive the benefits that come with fasting. With that said, each person is going to be different when it comes to fasting. They will need to follow different methods and may find that one method works better than another.

In order to maintain an intermittent fast, you need to consider which method is the best for you. It is fine to experiment a little bit in the beginning and see what works the best for you. If you find that alternate day fasting is too difficult for you, then it is fine to work with one of the other methods. All of them can be successful, you just have to give them the time they deserve.

In addition, you must make sure that you still feed your body adequate amounts of nutrition through the day. Yes, you are limiting the amount of time that you are allowed to eat, but this doesn't mean that you should go into a big calorie deficit or miss out on some important nutrients and minerals along the way. For some people, fasting can make them feel less hungry and they start cutting their calories too much. At least in the beginning you may want to consider tracking your calories to figure out whether or not you are taking in enough in your diet. Since intermittent fasting can, after the first few weeks, take away a bit of your hunger, you may be surprised at how few calories you consume and that you need to up it a bit more.

Eating healthy, sticking with the right number of calories and nutrients that the bod needs, and sticking with a version of the fast that you can actually enjoy are all the best tips that you can use to make sure that you can maintain an intermittent fasting lifestyle.

Consider Cutting Down Workouts and Adjusting the Hours

In the beginning, you will encounter numerous challenges especially coping with hunger and working out. This is because your body is not yet used to this lifestyle. However, you should not give up. Instead, think about making appropriate adjustments. For instance, you may go for walks instead of jogging. This way, you will manage to handle the challenges experienced during the initial stages.

Rest assured that your energy levels will get back to normal once this transition period is over. You will then realize that you can work harder than you did before. In the beginning, though, your limbs will feel weak, and you might lack the motivation to workout. Your hunger pangs will also rise. Learn to persevere and be strict with your eating window. It will be a good idea if this eating window comes right after your workout sessions.

You can adjust your workouts so that you start earlier or later than usual. Many people prefer their workouts to be within their fasting window to distract from the hunger. Others need to get the workouts scheduled to time the end of the fasting window, so they do not suffer from hunger afterward. Your workouts should be timed to suit your preferences, schedule, and priorities.

Consider the Use of Delayed Gratification

Delayed gratification is a simple process that works great when you start fasting. Consider a little child who asks its mom permission to go to the playground to play with other kids. Instead of a direct yes, the mother is likely to delay the approval to a later moment. The delay eases the pain of desire. You can consider delayed gratification as an excellent tool to help you handle your intermittent fasting lifestyle especially when you start feeling hungry.

In the course of each day, you are likely to be offered a snack by co-workers or see the delicious cereal and milk your child, or family member is eating. Your mouth may water and your heart filled with the desire to eat. Using the delayed gratification tactic, you can promise yourself the treat, not at that moment though but at a later time. You can consider putting this down on a piece of paper or diary to remind yourself how strong you are and how far you have come.

Re-organize your Meals

It is a good idea to consider rearranging your meals just so that you eat your complex carbs and protein first. Your list needs to contain foods such as vegetables, fruits, lean meat, fish, grains, and other healthy options. Choose foods that are high in nutrients to nourish your body adequately.

Try and organize your meals ahead of time. When you prepare your meals, remember to include a complex carbohydrate and protein. It is possible that by the time you get to your eating window, you will be hungry enough, so a ready meal after working out is always welcome. The order of your meals should first be proteins, followed by complex carbs, then simple carbs, and finally any delayed gratification foods.

Exercise while Fasting

You can also try out exercising during the fasting window. Working out during your fasting period is common with most women as they can burn more calories this way. Exercising during your fasting window is sometimes referred to as fasted training. You can try it and see if it works out for you. If not, then you can workout during your eating window.

When you workout during your fasting window, your insulin levels will be low. This means your body will not derive energy from the food that you eat but from stored fat. There are plenty of women who prefer working out on empty due to inherent benefits like the ability to burn more body fat. This helps to get rid of stubborn fat stored in the body.

Take a Before Photo

One other thing you may want to consider is taking a before photo. While it is not an essential aspect of intermittent fasting, it can provide a great reference point especially if one of your goals is to lose weight. Having these photos taken will help keep you motivated. You can continue taking photos after a couple of weeks into the fast to observe and note any significant changes.

Taking a before and after photo will help you monitor progress, especially if you are trying to lose belly fat or build muscle. As you fast, and workout, your body releases more HGH or human growth hormone. This hormone will help your body to develop lean, toned muscles over time. A progress photo will serve as an excellent motivation tool that will help you to keep focused on your weight loss goals.

The Bottom Line

What you need to keep in mind is that intermittent fasting is one of the most effective and successful lifestyle changes you will ever make in your life. However, getting started is the most challenging part. As a matter of fact, the first 10 days to 2 weeks will probably be the toughest yet. The good thing is that once you get used the lifestyle, you will easily get used to it and begin to enjoy the benefits shortly thereafter. You will be shocked at the drastic decrease in the cravings that you currently have, especially for junk foods and fast food.

Chapter 7: Sustaining Your New Regimen

Now that you started intermittent fasting and what you can expect from it as a woman, you will also want to know how to sustain your new regimen. There are things that can help with sustaining your diet, which you will want to do. Practicing intermittent fasting can be a complete lifestyle change because so much time suddenly becomes available. Therefore, you will want to practice things like forming new and better habits, putting the thing in place to hold yourself accountable, setting short and long-term goals, and keeping the right mindset. Later on, you can reference the **"Tips and Tricks"** section for a quick reference.

Differentiating Between Physiological Hunger and Psychological Hunger

It is true that there are actually two different ways you can feel hungry but only one is meant for proper functioning and survival or your body. They do both have important roles but psychological hunger, when blindly followed, can lead to the array of problems we can associate with overeating. However, to understand psychological hunger, you have to understand why we love food so much.

Obviously, we need food to survive and our food choices can determine whether we thrive or not. Nevertheless, why do we generally love all foods in their own ways, from apples to pasta? It is because when we consume foods, there is an increase in **dopamine production** in our brain. Dopamine is a neurotransmitter, something used by neurons to send signals between one another. The brain has existing dopamine pathways with some being directly linked to the way dopamine affects our motivation and the reward center of the brain. Whenever you feel happy about something happening, it is typically dopamine being released. Dopamine is released from small events to very large ones, like finding your keys, winning the lottery and sex. The things we consume also directly affect it and one of the main reasons recreation drugs work. However, food also makes us release dopamine, and certain types can make us release more or less. When you consume foods high in processed sugar, for example, it will result in significantly larger levels of dopamine being released and produced. The same goes for foods high in any kind of fat. It is one theory that our brains have not "caught up" evolutionarily to our caloric scarcity. A mere few-several hundred years ago food was extremely more scare than it is today, and before that even more, this may have been a driving factor in the way our brains reacted to calorically dense foods. Foods high in sugar and fat are extremely calorie dense, despite many being nutritionally deficient, and this might be a biological reason why they can be so hard to give up.

Psychological hunger is not only brought on by dopamine production but other issues/dysfunctions can bring on 'false' hunger signals as well. Your **thyroid** has a big say when it comes to your **appetite**. This gland is small and butterfly-shaped found in the neck and wrapped around your windpipe. This gland is responsible for extracting the iodine found in foods and creating hormones called T3 and T4. (36) These hormones directly affect your metabolism and can determine the speed and efficiency your bodily process functions. (36) The thyroid gland depends on signals from the pituitary gland but many things can interfere with these signals, things like environmental factors and diet. Depending on how these signals are disrupted, it can lead to two thyroid diseases known as **hyper**thyroidism and **hypo**thyroidism. If you have hyperthyroidism, your bodily process can be working in overdrive and your appetite can be stimulated when there is no real need for energy consumption. On the other hand, an underactive thyroid can do the opposite. Because you may feel hungry but do not actually need food, thyroid problems would fall in the category of psychological hunger.

Physiological hunger is when your body is in a real need of calories, blood sugar and or specific nutrients. When you are consuming food and thus driving insulin production, you can reach a threshold and the insulin will then reach the brain. Recent studies have shown that when insulin makes its way to your brain, it can stimulate appetite suppression and hinder hunger. This may be a natural hormonal and neurological way of your body telling you that it is full.

During the first few weeks of your journey, you will more than likely have to combat physiological hunger pains. A great way to do this is through distraction and deception. You can lie to your hunger receptors into feeling a sense of satiety with some simple tricks. If your fasting method involves you skipping breakfast, for instance, it will be helpful to not only drink a caffeinated beverage but also drink sparkling water. The carbonation in sparkling water works amazingly in bringing on a false sense of fullness. They are also typically supplemented with loads of beneficial minerals and vitamins that will help keep you healthy during a fast.

Once you know a little bit more about your hunger signals, you can make your own scale from 1-4 to rate how hungry you are. Then you can treat anything from 0-2 as psychological hunger and 2.1-4 as physiological hunger, with 0 being not hungry at all and 4 being full-blown physiological hunger.

Exercise

Exercise is a crucial aspect of any healthy lifestyle. All forms of exercise are amazing for your body including hormonal processes and nutrient efficiency, but some are better for targeting fat loss. If you are exercising or planning to, consider doing resistance training and high-intensity interval training (HIIT). Resistance training and HIIT is a great way to burn fat because they keep your heart rate within specific parameters known as the "fat-burning zone." The fat burning zone is when you maintain your rate at approx. 70-85% of your maximum heart rate. You can calculate your own heart rate by placing two fingers where your neck meets your jaw and feeling your pulse. Once you feel the heartbeat, start a 20-second timer and count how many beats occur. Make sure you have allowed yourself to reach a resting heart rate before you start measuring. Also, avoid letting your thumb touch as most people can feel their pulse through their thumb. Once you have counted, multiply that number by three and you will have your resting heart rate per minute. Once you know this, you can calculate 70-85% of this by

Intermittent Fasting For Women

multiplying your resting heart rate by .7 or .85. You can use the formula below for a quick reference.

Despite the slightly intimidating name, anyone can perform high-intensity interval training because intensity is a relative term in regards to exercise. This type of training involves you maintaining a slightly elevated heart rate with periods of explosive ATP energy being used, typically in quick sprints. For example, you can you can do a light jog and keep your heart rate at around 70% it's maximum for 45 seconds, followed by 15 seconds of maximum intensity and performance. Then repeat. Typically, this cycle is repeated for a total of 10-15 minutes and is widely used by professional athletes who want to improve cardio function and not lose muscle mass. Because the high-intensity period is so short, you have no excuse not to give it your best!

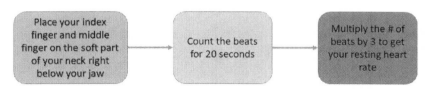

So, how should exercise be integrated into our unique regimen? Well, you will want to plan for days/times you will be fasting and days/times when you will be eating. As mentioned before, the time you eat things like carbohydrates can have significant effects on how the energy entering the body is treated. If your goal is to lose body fat, then after a workout, you are going to want to refrain from eating for at least 120 minutes. In this time, it is extremely important to stay hydrated and I recommend taking a multivitamin along with a branch-chained amino acid supplement. These supplements often come formulated for this very purpose so they contain zero carbohydrates or fats and many of them are less than 1 calorie per serving. Taking these steps when fasting after exercise is very important to ensure blood sugar levels do not drop dangerously low, you do not experience threatening light-headedness, or your hormonal process is not significantly disrupted.

Consuming protein after a workout will also reduce muscle soreness and improve muscle repair, branch chain amino acids are the building blocks of protein, so these supplements can be a great aid to have in your regimen. There will be certain days where certain exercises will be more beneficial towards your progress and health. On fasted days, try to keep the exercise at a low intensity or at a high intensity for a very short period, in order for you to avoid depleting yourself completely of your glycogen stores. On the other hand, days where you are eating more food, include higher intensity or longer workout sessions that burn more calories to prevent any significant storage of the energy you consumed that day. The table below is an example of an exercise plan integrated with a crescendo fasting method.

Example Workout Plan Integrated with a Crescendo Fasting Method

Example Workout Plan Integrated with a Crescendo Fasting Method							
	Mon	**Tues**	**Wed**	**Thur**	**Fri**	**Sat**	**Sun**
Fed or Fasted	Primarily fed day	Primarily fasted	Primarily fed day	Primarily fasted	Primarily fed day	Primarily fasted	Primarily fed day
Exercise Type	High volume resistance training	Yoga	High-intensity interval training	Rest day	Strength oriented	Yoga	High-intensity interval training

If your goal is to lose weight, then you will want to do certain t, then you will want to do certain types of exercise over others. Using techniques like HIIT will help you burn fat as a main result of it.

Count the amount of calories that you need

Ideally you will want to be sure to consume a majority of your daily caloric intake in the period immediately following your workout period. This will not only make it easier for your body to generate lean muscle mass it will also make it easier to recover from the workout. In order to do this, you are going to want to start by determining the caloric requirements your body needs in order to build muscle.

To do so, you are going to need to determine your basal metabolic rate (BMR) which is the number of calories you burn while resting. The more lean muscle mass you have, the higher your BMR is going to be. Essentially what this means is that the more muscular physique you have, the more calories you are going to be burning around the clock. The average human body burns about 60 percent of its daily calorie consumption just through natural daily processes. From there, the body burns about 30 percent of its energy on physical activity and 10 percent on digestion.

To determine how many calories your body burns while resting, you can use the following formula. First you will need to determine your weight in kilograms by dividing your current weight by 2.2. You will also need to determine your height in centimeters which can be found by taking your height in inches and multiplying by 2.54.

For women, your BMR is going to be equal to (65.09 + (9.56 x weight in kilograms) + (1.84 x height in centimeters) – (4.67 x Age).

The end result is the number of calories you burn while your body is at rest. For example, for a man who weighs 200 lbs. their BMR would be about 2,200 calories. From there, you are going to want to use the Sterling-Pasmore Equation to determine how many calories you need based on your current amount of lean body mass. Each pound of lean muscle mass requires 13.8 calories to support it. You can determine your current lean body mass from standard body fat measurements.

Calculate lean muscle mass vs. fat mass:

Body fat % x scale weight= fat mass

Scale weight - fat mass= lean body mass

Once you have determined your BMR, you will want to account for the additional calories that are burned through exercise.

- If you live a primarily sedimentary lifestyle you will want to multiply your BMR by 1.2.
- If you perform a light exercise routine 3 or 4 times per week you you will want to multiply your BMR by 1.375.
- If you perform moderate exercise between 3 and 5 days per week you will want to multiply your BMR by 1.55.
- If you exercise at a moderate intensity 6 or 7 days a week you will want to multiply your BMR by 1.725.

- If you are extremely active and exercise 6 or 7 days a week for 90 minutes or more you will want to multiply your BMR by 1.9.

With your BMR in mind, you are then going to want to consume about 20 percent of those calories before you exercise for the best results. This meal or snack should be a quality mix of both carbs and protein. Then, when you are finished exercising you are going to want to consume about 60 percent of your total calories sometime in the next 2 to 4 hours. This might seem like a lot but if you focus on calorie dense foods it should not be a problem.

Additionally, with this type of setup it is important to keep in mind that you are typically better off focusing on a diet with more carbs and less fat to support muscle growth. This is due to the fact that, following a workout, you are going to want to focus on carbs instead of fats which can be detrimental. This does not mean you are going to want to eliminate all fats, it just means you are going to want to limit the number of fats you consume in your post-workout meals.

If you lead a mostly sedimentary lifestyle then you will want to take in about 31 calories per kilogram per day to maintain your weight. If you are a recreational athlete then this number will be between 33 and 38 calories. If you are an endurance athlete then this number will be between 35 and 50 calories based on your training. If you are strength training and exercising heavily then this will be between 30 and 60 calories based on your training.

If you are looking to build muscle mass then you are going to want to ensure that you take in an additional 250 to 500 calories per day depending on the type of exercise you are doing. On the other hand, if you are exercising on a daily basis and are looking to lose weight then you should subtract an additional 300 calories from your daily intake. This will help you to not only lose weight, but also to maintain muscle mass in the process.

Habits

We all have bad habits, some worse than others. Breaking a habit can be a hard thing to do so it is usually better to replace them with better alternatives at first and gradually work your way from there. Bad habits can actually be considered a neurological dysfunction because they are intrusions of deceptive messages that can cause a load of problems. (31) These *deceptive messages* can result in someone engaging in unhealthy stress relievers and "reverting back to past. The beautiful thing about IF is if your goal is to lose weight, many of your portion sizes can remain the same, because you are mainly redirecting your body's energy sources by periodically restricting yourself from eating. According to Rebecca Gladding, M.D., co-author of the book, "You Are Not Your Brain," this may be one of the reasons why it is so hard to break bad habits successfully.

Depending on the habit you are trying to break, you can take a variety of different approaches. You can try replacing some habits with slightly healthier ones in some cases. For instance, if you happen to be a smoker, the number one successful approach to quitting is transitioning to vaping. A 10-year study done in the UK has determined that vaping is approximately 95% less harmful than smoking tobacco. A similar approach is taken in some rehabilitation programs in extreme cases, for instance heroin addicts are often given a substance called methadone to help them ween off the more harmful "habit." Other habits can be broken more slowly. If you have a bad soda pop habit, you can try replacing one a day with a healthier low sugar juice or a carbonated water.

In regards to food, we are kind of lucky in this day and age because there are so many delicious and healthy alternatives readily available in almost every supermarket. We now already know how to cut out saturated fat and cholesterol, but what about sugary treats and snacks? Readily available and delicious they are too good for some people to pass up, but maybe that is because they don't know of the other things they could get. Fruit is going to be your best friend here. Juicy, ripe sweet fruit packed with nutrients will give you a healthy sugar rush when you are in need. If your intermittent fasting method includes a morning meal, I highly recommend including a hefty portion of fruit in there to start your day.

Holding Yourself Accountable

Holding yourself accountable during your regimen is extremely important. Especially in regard to your nutritional and time parameters you have given to yourself. Disrupting the middle of a fast, the energy you consume may not even be used because insulin is already actively using the glycogen in your liver so it will then just be stored adding to weight gain. In simpler terms, your body will be too busy to use the food you eat as energy and then just store it for later. It is stored for later as fat. If it does end up converted into instant energy, it is less of an issue, yet it still temporarily destabilizes your insulin levels that could hurt the overall results your fasting has on your insulin sensitivity. (21)

There are many ways to hold yourself accountable. Keeping track of your nutrition is already one of them. By doing this, you are able to see clearly the numbers from day to day and week to week thus you can see an unbiased record of your actual progress. You can also incentivize yourself with rewards. Rewards are a great way for you to stay motivated and reach your goals. For instance, you could promise yourself a treat like your favorite snack, meal or restaurant at the end of every week as long as you stay within **your** preset guidelines. The beauty of these self-bettering practices is that there will literally be no incentive for you to cheat or lie to yourself, making it more likely you will succeed. If you mess up, there is no real embarrassment either because no one else has to know. Just be honest with yourself and move on from any mistakes.

Setting Long and Short-Term Goals

Formal goal setting is a good idea if you are serious about your destination. If your goal is to lose weight, then set a date and a specific weight you want to be by that date. Do this both long and short term. For your **long-term goals,** think in the timeline of 3, 6, 12 months, and beyond. Visualizing yourself succeeding can be a great way to stay motivated during your journey. If your goal is to lose weight, for instance, picture in your mind how you will look, and much more importantly feel when you get to where you want to be.

A 1,000-mile journey begins with a single step. Think of your **short-term goals** like mini milestones you reach on a daily basis. You will want to think of your short-term goals in terms of days and weeks. Your daily goals can involve things like achieving your base levels, getting in your required exercise, successfully meal prepping or many more. You will probably have a lot more daily goals than you will long-term goals so it can be helpful to make a list of your next days' goals the night before. Then schedule check-ins with yourself in periods like daily, every other day, and weekly. If you mess up on a daily goal, do not worry. The point of intermittent fasting is to give you control in the maintenance of your weight and insulin production in the long term. One mistake will not hinder as much progress as you think but not learning from that mistake can just be destructive.

You also want to set reasonable goals for yourself. Do not attempt or expect to lose 10 pounds per week safely for instance. That is not what intermittent fasting is about. Remember, when it comes it to intermittent fasting and women, it is an art!

Make sure to physically write your goals down or put them on your phones' home screen. Somewhere where you can always see them and be reminded about them. Goal setting can actually give you a significantly higher chance of success especially when you write them down. This is because writing them down put these goals deeper in your head and allows your subconscious to help you through your journey. (32)

Keeping the Right Mindset

This is the single most important psychological aspect you need to have during your journey. Intermittent fasting, especially at first, can require a lot of willpower and focus. Dr. Westie, who I mentioned in Chapter 2, found that in the first few weeks, there would definitely be mood changes. This is because of the sudden drops in blood sugar levels, they are not dangerous drops, but your body is still not used to them nonetheless. The brain actually functions of blood sugar so the changes can bring on some of these effects temporarily; anxiety, depression, edginess, and discomfort. For reference, the brain is basically the last thing that stops using glucose in the process of starvation, so the levels of glucose depletion you will be experiencing will be minimal in comparison. With the right mindset, however, you can combat these symptoms significantly.

It is good practice to keep yourself positive by writing down things every day and that you are close to accomplishing. If you make a mistake in a day, write it down and then think of a solution to write down. This can leave you reassured that you know how to proceed from the last hiccup.

Keep Busy

One thing you will for sure notice while you are intermittent fasting is the amount of extra time you have in the day or week! Think about how much of your day right now you spend thinking or doing something about your next meal. There is the cooking, the cleaning, the shopping and worst of all there is the deciding! With many intermittent fasting variations, you may be having 1-2 meals on your fasted day, and if you decide to prep, there will be even less work.

In your free time, try picking up a new habit or project. Meditation is an amazing thing to try if you do not already. Meditation can help maintain your positive mindset, lets you reflect on your progress honestly, and calm your mind from the busy lives we all live today. All you need to meditate too is 15 minutes and a quiet place. Surround yourself with the thing that brings you peace like your favorite comfy at home outfit, a warm coffee beverage, and your favorite relaxing music, preferably something instrumental. Set a time, forget about it, and allow your mind to be in the moment with no distraction. Practicing this on a daily basis can bring on loads of psychological benefits and thus physiological benefits as well.

Keeping your mind active is also important. Once you have passed the transition page, look for a project or subject that interests you, one that takes a greater level of thinking and time. You can also get in the habit of tracking your progress in your respective projects while you also track your weight-controlling journey with intermittent fasting. Getting in the habit of being honest with yourself and tracking the progress you make in all aspects of life while also rewarding yourself for successfully doing so can really help with motivating you to achieve further goals.

Drink Coffee

Tea works too but there is 50-70% more of the active appetite suppressing ingredient in coffee. You can also take it in pill form if you are concerned about specific dosing and obtaining the perfect amount for you. The ingredient caffeine will really help you with appetite suppression and will make it much easier for you to go without food, especially at first. (35)

Caffeine is a stimulant and does not directly suppress appetite. Instead, it actually is directing the body to use its sympathetic nervous system (fight or flight) which lowers the energy directed at digestive functions.

Caffeine also stimulates thermogenesis in your body. Do you remember early on in chapter 4 when I mentioned celery and how it does not actually burn calories? Well, coffee has a stimulating effect on the process of heat production in your body, that process is thermogenesis. While coffee still does not burn calories within itself, the thermogenic effect of its consumption paired with exercise and fasting can further increase the energy into heat production.

While caffeine consumption will be a greatly beneficial aid, especially for newcomers to intermittent fasting, when sourced from coffee and tea it can also have dehydrating effects. The caffeine in coffee increases blood flow to the liver and makes your body excrete more fluids than consumed. This is why when you drink a lot of coffee or a sugary drink like iced tea, you will find yourself making frequent trips to the washroom. Because it is extremely important to stay hydrated during any fasting journey, it can be safe practice to limit yourself to two cups of coffee per day on fasting days, and one on another day. You can also correlate how much water you drink with how much coffee you had. Meaning, you can drink two glasses of water for every cup of coffee you drink. Beware however, of this method, you may find yourself running to the ladies' room every 15 minutes, and too much peeing can flush you of all your electrolytes which play important roles in brain function especially while fasting.

Find Support in Your Community

You may need to search online for some forums, talk to your family and friends, and actively seek like-minded individuals on a daily basis. Even before you start your fast, you can talk to people who are experienced in the area or whose opinions you value. You can tell them about your plans and even see if they are willing to give you feedback. While you actually are intermittent fasting, the internet and social media can be an amazing source to find support with any issue you might run into. If you stay up to date in the community, you will also become aware of new research coming out, be able to learn from other peoples' mistakes, and prevent yourself from making mistakes in the first place as well. There are also a plentiful number of professional athletes and people of interest you can follow through social media to learn more and more on a daily basis. The more you surround yourself with experts on intermittent fasting, the more you will eventually know.

Build Your New Regimen Around Your Existing Life

While you plan out your intermittent fasting, keep in mind the times of day and days of the week you like to socially eat and drink. If you typically go out after work on Fridays for example, and you are using the crescendo fasting method, make sure a feeding day is going to line up with Fridays. All of us live busy lives and you do not want intermittent fasting to make you miserable. It is supposed to be a positive lifestyle change. So if you are in your journey already and finding more and more social roadblocks every day, consider changing the form of your plan. On the other hand, if you are facing numerous roadblocks on a daily basis, it may be an indication you need to eliminate some unhealthy habits from your life. Remember your health is the most important thing, not your social life.

Another way you can mitigate your social life and fasting regimen from clashing is to become **adaptive.** Learn to adapt on the spot to spontaneous social situations. Someone's birthday at work and they offered you cake on a fasted day? Say thank you and take it home for your reward at the end of the week. On a fed day? See if it can potentially fit into your macros for the day without you eliminating any beneficial components of that day's food.

Chapter 8: Interm DEBUNKED Fasting Myths

Now that we have covered the science and history, benefits, how you as a woman should take extra precaution, and who should not practice intermittent fasting, let's debunk some common myths you may have heard about it. This section will contain the information you can use to quickly rebuttal any common criticisms people may throw at you. If you look online, you will see an endless supply of content preaching misinformation on almost every subject. Intermittent fasting is no different. Here some myths you should know are not true.

MYTH: "You should NEVER be intermittent fasting if you're a woman. You'll mess up all your hormones!"

While intermittent fasting as a woman may take a few extra precautions, it is a perfectly safe practice for most women. While some methods practiced may seem harsh, proper practice will only benefit hormonal processes. You are controlling the trends of insulin production within your own body and thus controlling how much energy is used by your intake of calories and your previously stored energy (glycogen).

If you are an athlete, for instance, a bodybuilder, and in the stage of increasing your muscle mass, then less intense variations of the crescendo method are what you should star with. Also, try consuming many healthy calories dense foods peanut butter is an amazing source of protein, good fats, and calories!

MYTH: "Intermittent fasting lets you lose fat while bulking up."

In most cases, intermittent fasting is usually a weight loss treatment and prevention, however, if you are into maintaining your bodyweight while resistance training, you will need to take a different approach by eating many more calories in your feeding windows. However, if your goal is to lose weight, then intermittent fasting will naturally have you in a caloric deficit You cannot gain weight while in a true calorie deficit because this means you are expelling more energy than you are consuming. If you could gain weight while in a deficit, it would mean you could create something out of nothing. Therefore, you will not lose fat and gain muscle at the same time.

MYTH: "You will lose too much muscle if you practice intermittent fasting."

While it would be very unlikely for you to gain weight while intermittent fasting when done properly, there shows no significant muscle mass reduction. For the average woman, once you have transitioned to a fast, your body will then start to use the glycogen previously stored in your liver. Following your liver fat cells, the glycogen found in your other fat cells will be used for energy. The body basically only uses carbohydrates and fats as energy, protein is an extremely inefficient source and thus will only start to be used at the beginning of the starvation process. [4]

MYTH: "If you intermittent fast, no matter what, you will become malnourished."

This is false. The average woman aged 18-60 needs 200-2,400 calories per day to maintain their body weight. An appropriately formed meal plan will be designed to deliver you a minimum of 2-5% above your own calculated base levels.

MYTH: "Intermittent fasting is just an alternative to snacking all day long"

This is far from the case. While limiting yourself to **healthy** snacks and not full meals all day, you most likely will be in a caloric deficit and thus lose weight, however, it will have no benefit on your insulin sensitivity. If the snack you consume isn't clean and not quality ingredients, then this will actually contribute to your insulin resistance.

Chapter 9: Weight Loss, Lean Body, and Getting the Best Body of Your Life

Many people who go on an intermittent fast are doing it as a way to help them get leaner, trimmer, and lose weight. They are tired of getting stuck in plateaus, or they are ready to start their weight loss journey for good and have decided that intermittent fasting is the right choice for them to reach this goal. If you are on an intermittent fast in order to lose weight, then this chapter is for you. We will discuss some of the keys to maintaining and losing weight, how to exercise the right way, why muscle gain is good for this weight plan, and so much more!

What are the biggest keys to weight loss and maintaining my weight loss?

There are a lot of tips out there that claim to be the best for helping you to lose weight, even though a lot of them tend to contradict themselves. One will promise weight loss if you do this, but then the next talks about how that original idea will just make you gain weight. When you are ready to use intermittent fasting to help you lose weight, then make sure to follow these important tips:

- Start with a healthy diet: A healthy diet is one of the most important things when it comes to weight loss. Sure, exercise is important and can help out with weight loss. But exercise is only about 20 percent of the story while the diet you eat is about 80 percent. Make sure that you are eating a well-balanced diet, and weight loss will be easier than before.

- Watch your portions: This is especially important right when you end your fast. You are going to feel very hungry after the fast, and may want to just gobble up everything in sight. But you need to be mindful of your portions to ensure that you don't take in too much even after the fast.

- Try mindful eating: Too many times, we get a plate of food in front of us, and we just scarf it down as quickly as possible. By the time our stomach can tell the brain that it is full, we have taken in way too many calories and weight lass is lost. Mindful eating is when you take your time, think through what you are eating, slowly chew your bites, and learn how to listen to your body. When you eat in this manner, you ensure that the body gets enough calories, but you can stop in plenty of time before going overboard and eating too much.

- Avoid emotional triggers: Emotional triggers can cause even the best laid plans to get ruined. If you eat because you are bored, when you are tired, when you feel upset, or for any other reasons other than hunger, then this can be a big problem. You need to learn how to avoid or handle these emotional triggers to ensure that you see the weight loss that you deserve.

- Don't drink the calories: Remember that you shouldn't drink up the calories that you need during the day. A coffee with some extras here, a little soda there, some wine with supper, and more can quickly add up. They may not be worth a lot of calories on their own, but when you combine all of those and more into your day, you are taking in a lot of extra calories, without any of the extra nutritional benefits. Try to stick mostly to water, tea, coffee, and other non-caloric beverages and keep your calories reserved for high-quality and nutritious foods.

- Have a goal in mind: When you have a good goal in mind and you keep your motivation high, you are going to see weight loss with any type of diet plan. Write out the goal and leave it somewhere that you can see on a regular basis. This will ensure that you can see the great results that you want, without feeling down or giving up.

How to experience weight loss in a safe and effective way

While an intermittent fast can be a great way to help you to naturally limit the number of calories that you consume each day, it is also important to have a good idea of how many calories you should take in each day, and how many you would need to cut off in order to help you lose weight and feel your best. Each person is going to be different and often figuring out your goals, how much you need to lose, and how quickly you would like to lose it can determine how much of a calorie deficit you need.

First, we need to calculate the amount of calories that you need just to survive each day. This is an essential number that can help you maintain, gain, or lose weight based on your goals. Often the Harris-Benedict formula is going to be used to help determine your basal metabolic rate. This rate is going to be determined by a few different factors including your body size, age, and sex. This number is simply going to tell you how many calories that you would burn up just being awake and alive. Of course, since even on lazy days you get out of bed and move around some, there need to be some adjustments to the number. Let's look at the basic formula for this one first thought.

For women, the formula is 655 + (4.35 X weight in pounds) + (4.7 X height in inches) − (4.7 X age in years)

This is just the number that you need if you just woke up and stayed in bed all day long. In addition, you will need to come up with a new number based on how active you are each day. the numbers that you can use include:

- Sedentary or little to not exercise during the week: 1.2
- Lightly active or you workout lightly for a few days a week: 1.375
- Moderately active or you workout at a moderate pace three to five days a week: 1.55
- Very active or you do hard exercise and work 6 to 7 days of the week: 1.725
- Extra active: 1.9

Determine your activity level and then multiply it with the BMR that you got in the first formula. This will give you the number of calories that you need just to maintain your current weight. Be honest with yourself here. If you just go on a few light walks after supper, ten it is probably best to keep yourself at sedentary rather than at lightly active. If you pick an activity level higher than your current one, you are just harming yourself.

From here, you need to work on a calorie deficit in order to actually lose weight. You can do this with adding in some more exercise, while maintaining the same food intake, or by lowering your calories each day. Doing a combination of both often works out well for most people. This helps them to not fee too deprived when they are going without food, and then you don't have to workout like crazy to maintain it either. Some of the ways that you can limit your calories and end up with a deficit at the end of the day include:

- For optimal weight loss, you will want to reduce your calories to about 15 to 20 percent below the maintenance levels we have above.
- You should reduce your calories by about 500, but never more than 1000.

- For women, it is best to not go below 1200 calories during the day. Going too much below this on a regular basis can be hard to maintain and will make it difficult to get the nutrition that you need.
- It is best to aim for about 10 to 2 pounds of weight loss each week. If you are losing weight a lot faster than this, then it is unlikely that you are losing fat.

Should I focus on weight loss or fat loss?

There can be a big difference when it comes to losing fat and losing weight. Your goal with a fast should be to concentrate more on losing fat, rather than weight. When you lose weight, you may lose a bit of everything, including organ size, fluids, muscle, and fat. But with fat loss, you are just concentrating on losing fat, and none of the other stuff. When you lose fat, you will lose weight, you are just concentrating that weight loss on strictly losing fat, rather than losing all the other stuff as well.

To help you determine whether you are just losing weight or if you are losing fat, you can do a body fat test. If you are a female who is about 150 pounds with 35 percent fat, then you are carrying over 52 pounds of fat on the body. An ideal healthy woman will be around 25 percent fat, which means 37 pounds (if we go with the 150 pound woman), so a loss of 15 pounds of fat would be helpful for getting her at a healthier level.

If you were just concentrating on losing weight, you may be able to lose 20 pounds total, but if only ten of those pounds can from the fat stores of the body, you would still be at 32 percent fat on the body. To reach the 25 percent body fat level in the example that we talked about before, all of the 20 pounds needs to come from fat.

When you are losing weight, the best way to lose just fat is to add in some strength training to the fitness plan you are doing. While cardio can help you temporarily lose some fat and can be good for your heart, the pounds you lose from this type of exercise will just come back when you stop or limit the cardio. This is because you aren't building up muscle mass to help get the weight up. Many women are worried about bulking up when they do weight lifting, or gaining on too much muscle. This isn't really a concern for most of the population so it is fine to add in some weight training to increase muscle throughout the body.

Many people on an intermittent fast worry that they either have to lose fat or gain muscle, that they aren't able to do both. But these two ideas aren't exclusive and you can see some benefits from both working together. When you implement a weight lifting routine into your life, even if it is just for a few days a week, you are going to quickly notice that there is more fat loss, that you trim up, and that it is easier to burn through the calories than ever before.

Now, when you lose weight, it is unavoidable to sometimes lose weight from other sources than fat. You want the majority to come from fat, but there is going to be some water weight and even muscle mass weight when you focus on losing weight over all. But with the loss of muscle mass, you may have a rebound effect that can lead to weight gain over time. Muscle is very active metabolically and it can light the furnace so that your metabolism is fast and will burn through calories. With the right amount of muscle mass, you will burn more calories, even if you just sit on the couch for the day. when you lose muscle mass, it means that the metabolism is going to slow down, and the weight will come back on.

If you are just focusing on weight loss, you are going to start losing some muscle mass. This is why it is so important to implement a weight lifting plan into your routine. Too many times we focus on just doing cardio to help with weight loss. Cardio can be important too and you shouldn't ignore it. But adding in at least a few days of weight lifting can make a difference when it comes to your workout and how much muscle mass you are able to keep.

Chapter 10: The Best Diet Plan to Complement an Intermittent Fast

When you decide to go on an intermittent fast, you will find that you can pick out any kind of diet plan that you want. There isn't an official diet plan out there for fasting and any of them can work. The important part is to remember that you need to eat healthy and wholesome foods. If you continue to eat your traditional diet with lots of sugars, carbs, and processed foods, there is no hope for you seeing great results with intermittent fasting.

With that said, many people have found that adding the ketogenic diet with an intermittent fast can be one of the best things to speed up their results and to help stave off hunger. Both of these diet plans focus on putting the body into ketosis, or the process where the body burns fat instead of carbs. A ketogenic diet is one that focuses on eating very low amounts of carbs during the day, usually under 50 grams for the whole day.

The rest of your calories will come from healthy fats and moderate amounts of protein.

On its own, an intermittent fast does amazing for helping you to lose weight and, while you are fasting, it can hep your body switch over to burning fat for fuel. But when you get to your eating window, it is possible to load up on carbs and then the body switches back to that as an energy source. You can still see results, but when you implement the ketogenic diet in as well, the body will never receive enough carbs to sue as a viable fuel source. The body will start to just rely on healthy fats for fuel.

Fat is a much more efficient form of energy than carbs and sugars can be. The body will be able to burn through the fats that you eat, as well as any excess body fat that is lying around and causing weight gain and health conditions. Many people find that adding both the ketogenic diet and an intermittent fast together can do some wonders for their overall health and can make them lose weight almost overnight.

The intermittent fasting part is going to work the same when you combine these two eating plans. You simply pick the method that works the best for you, and then stick with the protocol that works for it. With the ketogenic diet though, you will need to make some changes to the way that you eat.

The ideas of a ketogenic diet are pretty simple to follow, but they do turn traditional ideas about dieting upside down. With the ketogenic diet, you will focus on consuming high amounts of healthy fats, moderate amounts of protein, and very low amounts of carbs. About 70 to 75 percent of your calories a day should come from healthy sources of fat, like meats, cheeses, dairy, and olive oil. About 20 percent of your daily calories can come from a healthy source of protein. And the last five percent should be reserved for your carbs, mainly in the form of fresh product to give your body the nutrients it needs.

When you can combine these two eating plans together, the body then enters into ketosis faster than ever before. Ketosis helps the body to burn up a lot of extra fat around the body, can give you more energy, and will finally help you break your addiction to sugars and carbs in favor of healthier foods.

While you can technically pick out any kind of diet plan that you want when it comes to an intermittent fast, as long as it focuses on eating healthy and nutritious foods, many people find that going on the ketogenic diet along with an intermittent fast is one of the best ways to ensure that they stay healthy and lose weight as quickly as possible.

Chapter 11: Tips & Tricks

Use this section as a quick reference to the benefits of a well-planned and methodically executed intermittent fasting regimen provided to you as a woman.

How to Stay Motivated as You Fast

Most people start off any diet really motivated at the beginning but then get discouraged when they do not get the results they want fast enough. First, you need to understand that this is a lifestyle and not an overnight diet. You also need to understand that nothing is easy or instant. Everything takes a little time. Here are some tips that can help you stay motivated.

Take each day at a time, and Track Your Progress

It is important to track not just your daily progress but to avoid being too hard on yourself when you do not reach a given checkpoint. Think to this to yourself: how can I improve from here? Devise a step-by-step plan to get there. You can do this for the simplest of problems as practice and then implement this problem solving method in larger areas of your life. Write everything down and compare your past data to your current data regularly

Shop the Perimeter and Prepare Your Food

The healthier foods in grocery stores are typically on the perimeter of the store. Most processed foods are high in salt, sugar, fat, and cholesterol. Make it a habit to consume whole foods. Meal prepping will not only save you even more time, it will also make you more likely to stick to your plan. Make a habit of prepping your food 2-3 time per week.

Keep Your Body Guessing

Change up the exercises you do on a regular basis and follow a diet with lots of quality variety. Experts suggest that to avoid hitting a plateau in your work you should switch up your work-out routine every 2-5 weeks. Plateaus happens when your body starts adapting to an exercise routine. www.bodybuilding.com is an excellent resource to change up your work out.

Stay Hydrated!

This tip is basically the easiest of them all yet it is one of the most avoided. You need to drink a lot of water and other beverages throughout the day. Not everyone loves the taste of water or having to go to the bathroom every half an hour. Nevertheless, it is crucial to ensure that you are drinking as close to a gallon of water per day as possible because being in a fasted state will cause your body to become dehydrated faster than would otherwise be the case. What's more, drinking more water will actually cause you to feel more full, more regularly, making the fasting process easier as a result.

Even then, taking water frequently has its numerous benefits. One of these is to keep you satisfied, so you do not feel hungry most of the time. A lot of the time, the hunger we feel is often dehydration. It is therefore important that you drink lots of water and stay hydrated throughout the day.

Apart from water, you can also have a cup of tea or coffee. Even then, to remain hydrated, take water throughout the day. When you are without food in your system, the body takes the opportunity to detoxify the liver. The water you drink will be used to clear out the toxins. If you do not drink water, the toxins will be eliminated with reserve water in your body. This will leave you quite dehydrated.

141

Drink Bone Broth

Alternatively, you can drink bone broth when you are fasting. If you get bored of water and other beverages, then give bone broth a try. You can choose to prepare some at home or buy pre-packed at the local grocery store.

Broth contains very little calories which is negligible in our case. However, the benefits of the micronutrients in bone broth are immense. For many years, this broth has been acknowledged as an effective appetite suppressant. Studies confirm that it actually can suppress appetite in mammals. It is thought to have anti-obesity properties and is well known for regulating blood sugar.

Should hunger pangs persist as you fast, then heat one cup and consume. One cup is sufficient to suppress hunger and keep you satiated until time for your meal.

Consider enlisting professional support:

You should consult a health expert before fully embarking on this very beneficial lifestyle. A health expert can guide you through the changes you need to make and enable you to transition safely into the intermittent fasting lifestyle. You should consider seeking advice instead of trying to guess what is right for you.

How to Stay Motivated as You Fast

Most people start off any diet really motivated at the beginning but then get discouraged when they do not get the results they want fast enough. First, you need to understand that this is a lifestyle and not an overnight diet. You also need to understand that nothing is easy or instant. Everything takes a little time. Here are some tips that can help you stay motivated.

Use a mirror and not the scales

At the start of your diet, take a look at yourself after a shower. Observe your body closely and notice which parts need toning and where you need to lose some fat. You can also take a picture of yourself and keep observing changes on a regular basis. Avoid using a weighing scale because it is bound to discourage you.

Eat a variety of foods

Nobody enjoys eating the same food each day. You need to find out which are the best foods possible for fasting days and ensure to eat healthy on your free days. Once you get to discover great foods, you will be able to discover new recipes and how to prepare meals that you actually enjoy.

Start with a friend

When you start the intermittent fasting lifestyle, find someone you can partner with. It could be a partner, family member, spouse, or a close friend. Go through the diet with him/her and use each other as a coach when working out. You can also motivate and cheer each other up. Having someone to plan meals with and go grocery shopping with is a great way to stay motivated.

Even as you fast, remember to continue maintaining a healthy lifestyle. Learn to eat healthy foods and have a balanced diet always. Always choose fresh produce and unprocessed foods. If you get enough rest each day, workout regularly, and fast periodically, then you will soon be healthier, look better, lose weight, and enjoy all the benefits that come with intermittent fasting.

Stay Positive

A woman with a positive and goal-oriented mindset will be far more likely to succeed. During your intermittent fasting journey, remember that it is a catalyst for a lifestyle change and not intended to be an extremely restrictive or harsh diet. Exercise, intellect testing activities, spending time in nature, meditating and yoga are only some of the many ways you can take action to stay positive during your journey!

Chapter 12: Longer Fasts, Why Intermittent Fasting for Women is an Art and Wrapping Things Up

Once you have tried your hand at intermittent fasting received benefits and decided that this lifestyle and regimen are for you, you may also want to try a longer fast to see what benefits that can bring. It is important to be reasonable when you experiment with longer fasting methods and responds to any adverse effects you might experience immediately. Do not go starting your first long fast by trying to go for a full week, start with something like a full 48 hours. Fasting like this, while closer to extreme, is still a proven way to catalyze weight loss. After your body is sourcing a majority of its energy from your liver and fat cells, you can expect to start losing weight and a significantly rapid weight loss. This is because your body will be using your fat as energy instead.

Weight loss can average between 1 and 2 pounds per day for the first week or so and then gradually slowdown from there to an average of about half a pound per day. (37) This is mainly due to losing water weight, but it will also depend on a variety of individual factors. These long fasts will in a sense force your body into **ketosis,** the specific name for when your body is primarily using fat as energy. The longer you are in ketosis, the more fat-stores that will be used as energy. After the fast, if you decide to keep losing weight you may increase your intake of proteins while lowering your intake of fats. As said before however, fat intake should never drop below 15% of your nutritional portfolio to be safe for women.

While these longer fasts can be effective in significantly increasing weight loss and even be used to cleanse the body of toxin build up, it should be considered to more closely resemble a crash diet. One study in a postgraduate medical journal has 46 patients fast for a period of two weeks to study the effects on weight loss in a scientific setting. Of course, all patients who fasted correctly lost weight, but in the 2 years follow up, 50% of patients more than likely gained their weight back. [38]

It can be a lot to take in, I know, but we have now covered everything you need to know about intermittent fasting as a woman. While fasting, in general, is an effective weight loss tool, intermittent fasting is far more effective in not only losing weight but maintaining a healthy bodyweight afterward as well.

As a woman, intermittent fasting is an art. How so? If you take some of the history's great artists, for example, they all have some commonalities i.e. patience, determination, focus, perseverance, direction and a whole lot of trial and error. Chances are you will have some mess-ups on your intermittent fasting journey and that is okay! At first, think of it as an experiment by trying the different common methods and giving them your own unique tweaks. This part will take patience and focus. Keep track of your progress and results from the respective methods, be honest in your reflection of yourself and plan on how to improve. I wanted to explain intermittent fasting to you as a woman from a scientific perspective first to clarify any concerns you may have about health and wellness. With an oversaturation of fasting warnings for women online, most having no scientific basis and purely living off on rumor and hype, it is important to stay informed and know the basic biological processes that are actually affected by intermittent fasting. Finally, it takes direction. Once again, you must set goals for where you want to go and who you want to be in order to be successful in your journey. After all, a journey without a destination is really just wandering, wandering back and forth.

In conclusion, intermittent fasting for most women is more than a suitable tool for weight loss and healthy weight management. This is only true if the fasting regimen is well planned based on personal knowledge and when full of a diet free of saturated fats and cholesterol and a variety of healthy quality foods.

Terms and Definitions

Chapter 1

Fasted State: A metabolic state in which previously inaccessible fat stores are used as energy. Typically, this will take 12 hours of fasting to achieve or regular intermittent fasting over time.

Fasting: The process in which someone consciously restricts the calories consumed to a variety of individual parameter for a number of varying reasons i.e. weight loss and cultural practices

Fed State: A metabolic state achieved when higher levels of nutrients, blood sugar, and insulin are in the blood from a recent intake of calories.

Intermittent Fasting: Consciously restricting caloric intake and controlling insulin blood level on a regular and periodic basis.

Metabolism: The chemical process that is sensitive to hormonal and environmental factors, your body in-charge of energy consumption, production, and usage.

Obesity: Body fat percentages and excess belly fat have reached a threshold and adverse health effects are experienced. This is linked directly to the consumption of foods high in sugar, saturated fat, and dietary cholesterol.

Ramadan: A cultural practice of Muslims wherein they fast every day from dawn to dusk for a month.

Chapter 2

Autonomic Nervous System: The part of the nervous system that is responsible for all unconscious body processes. A biological process that you do not have to do consciously such as breathing and keeping your heart beating.

Diabetes: A disease that hinders the ability of the body to produce or even respond to insulin. This results in dangerously higher blood sugar levels and metabolic dysfunction.

Hypertension: The term used to describe abnormally high blood pressure

LDL Cholesterol and HDL Cholesterol: LDL or low-density lipoproteins are also known as bad cholesterol. When reading nutrition labels, the cholesterol listed on them will be LDL cholesterol. LDL is directly linked to heart disease, the number one killer worldwide. HDL or high-density lipoprotein is produced by the body and is able to combat the effects of LDL to some degree.

Microbes: A microscopic organism such as bacteria.

Saturated Fat: A type of fat in which its molecules are saturated and solid at room temperature. This fat is typically found in large amounts in meat and dairy products and is directly linked to heart disease as well as other life-threatening illness.

Sympathetic: This belongs to the autonomic nervous system and is involved in the fight or flight response.

Parasympathetic: This belongs to the autonomic nervous system and is involved with the bodily process including rest and digestion.

Chapter 3

Gonads: The sexual organ that produces gametes. Known as Ovaries in women and testis in men.

Hormones: These regulatory substances are involved with almost every biological process. Hormones are typically produced within your body and then travel through the blood to their respective cells but can also be synthesized and injected.

Hypothalamus: A part of the brain responsible for the automatic nervous system and the pituitary gland.

Insulin: A hormone created by the pancreas designed to manage the glucose levels in your blood. Insulin is a key hormone to know about when intermittent fasting as a woman.

Insulin Resistance: This is when your cells are responding abnormally to insulin. This puts you at a higher risk of diabetes and metabolic syndrome. Consistently high levels of insulin might possibly lead you to develop insulin resistance.

Insulin Sensitivity: A term used to describe the insulin ability to regulate incoming energy efficiently. People who are insulin sensitive will need less insulin to regulate glucose. Intermittent fasting aims to increase your insulin sensitivity.

Pituitary Gland: Directly instructed by the hypothalamus, this produces hormones that play important roles in body processes like metabolism, including thirst and hunger.

Chapter 4

Base Levels: Refers to the minimum amount of macronutrients, and more importantly calories, that you need in order for you not to get sick.

Caloric Intake/Output: Refers to the ratio of calories you consume and expand on a daily or weekly basis. If it is less than 1, you can expect to lose weight and if it is greater than 1, you can expect to gain.

Calories: A unit of energy. Specifically, in our diet, how much energy it takes for the temperature of 1 kilogram of water to rise by 1 °C

Carbohydrates: One of the three main macronutrients and the most efficient source of energy. One carbohydrate is approximately 4 calories.

Current Levels: The levels of macronutrients, calories, and physical activity you are getting on average in your daily life.

Desired Levels: These depend completely on you as an individual and your goals. Calculate your base levels and then formulate your desired levels reasonably.

Fats: One of the three macronutrients. There are three types of fats: trans, saturated, and unsaturated fats. One gram of fat is approximately 9 calories.

Iron: A vital micronutrient responsible for transporting oxygen in red blood cells. Healthy sources of iron will be dark green leafy vegetables and fortified plant-based milk.

Macronutrients: Nutrients needed in particularly large amounts. The three main macronutrients are protein carbohydrates and fats.

Monosaccharides: The simplest form of carbohydrates and sugars.

Omega-3 Fatty Acids: An unsaturated fatty acid essential in forming a healthy diet. Healthy sources include nuts and vegetable oils.

Polysaccharides: Complex molecules of carbohydrates.

Protein: One of the 3 macronutrients. This is most responsible for muscle repair and growth of body tissues. One gram of protein is approximately 4 calories.

Thermogenesis: The production of heat in a human or animal body

Trans Fats: A primarily industrially produced partially saturated fat. Trans fatty acids lead to an even high risk of heart disease, atherosclerosis, and other life-threatening illness.

Chapter 5

The 5:2 Method: Fasting method with an 8-hour eating window on 2 days a week while also restricting calories on these days to approximately 500 calories.

The 16:8 Method: Fasting method where food consumption is restricted within an eight-hour window and fasting for the remaining sixteen hours every day.

The 24-hour Method: Fasting method that involves you fasting for a twenty-four-hour period, one to two times per week.

Alternate Day Method: Fasting method where you can eat regularly every other day and practice a complete fast or restrict the other days to approximately 500 calories

Crescendo Method: The #1 recommended intermittent fasting method for women. Fasting method where you eat in 8-12 hour windows 4 days a week and fast for 12-16 hour windows 3 days per week.

Chapter 6

High-Intensity Interval Training: Method of training where you keep your heart rate at around 70% its maximum capacity for 45 seconds, followed by 15 seconds of maximum intensity and performance. Then repeat. Typically, this cycle is repeated for a total of 10-15 minutes.

High Volume Resistance Training: Form of resistance or weight training with lighter weight loads and higher numbers of sets and reps. This form of training is ideal for growth and size of skeletal muscles as well as increasing muscle endurance.

Strength-Oriented Resistance Training: Form of resistance or weight training where weight loads are heavier and testing your maximum capabilities. This form of training is typically gained towards gaining strength and stability.

Citation (APA style)

(1) Not, B. F., Sugar. (n.d.). Intermittent Fasting (Time-Restricted Eating). Retrieved October 6, 2018, from http://burnfatnotsugar.com/assets/if.pdf

(2) Seimon RV, Roekenes JA, Zibellini J, Zhu B, Gibson AA, Hills AP, Wood RE, King NA, Byrne NM, Sainsbury A. Do intermittent diets provide physiological benefits over continuous diets for weight loss? A systematic review of clinical trials. *Mol Cell Endocrinol.* 2015 Dec 15;418:153-72

(3) McCulloch, D., MD. (n.d.). How Insulin Works. Retrieved from https://wa.kaiserpermanente.org/healthAndWellness/index.jhtml?item=/common/healthAndWellness/conditions/diabetes/insulinProcess.html

(4) Cahill, G. F. (1965). Metabolic Fuels. *Anesthesia & Analgesia,44*(5). doi:10.1213/00000539-196509000-00001

(5) Li, L., Wang, Z., & Zuo, Z. (2013). Chronic Intermittent Fasting Improves Cognitive Functions and Brain Structures. Retrieved from https://www.ncbi.nlm.nih.gov/pmc/articles/PMC3670843/

(6) Kollias, H. (2018, February 23). Intermittent Fasting for women: Important information you need to know. Retrieved from https://www.precisionnutrition.com/intermittent-fasting-women

(7) U. (n.d.). Estimated Calorie Needs per Day by Age, Gender and Physical Activity Level. *USDA Food Patterns.* Retrieved from https://www.cnpp.usda.gov/sites/default/files/usda_food_patterns/EstimatedCalorieNeedsPerDayTable.pdf.

(8) Craig, W. J., Mangels, A. R., & American, A. S. (2009, July). Position of the American Dietetic Association: Vegetarian diets. Retrieved from https://www.ncbi.nlm.nih.gov/pubmed/19562864/

(9) Alberts, B. (1970, January 01). The Shape and Structure of Proteins. Retrieved from https://www.ncbi.nlm.nih.gov/books/NBK26830/#A410

(10) Carbohydrates. (n.d.). Retrieved from https://www.eufic.org/en/whats-in-food/article/the-basics-carbohydrates

(11) Rose, I. (n.d.). Types of Sugar : Monosaccharides and Disaccharides. Retrieved from http://www.ivyroses.com/HumanBiology/Nutrition/Types-of-Sugar.php

(12) A., & B. (2013, January 29). Nutrient timing revisited: Is there a post-exercise anabolic window? Retrieved from https://jissn.biomedcentral.com/articles/10.1186/1550-2783-10-5?TB_iframe=true&width=921.6&height=921.6

(13) Yahoo Health. (2014, September 07). Why Women Need to Hydrate Differently Than Men. Retrieved from https://www.yahoo.com/lifestyle/why-women-need-to-hydrate-differently-than-men-96701060353.html

(14) Kerndt, P. R., Naughton, J. L., Driscoll, C. E., & Loxterkamp, D. A. (1982, November). Fasting: The History, Pathophysiology and Complications. Retrieved from https://www.ncbi.nlm.nih.gov/pmc/articles/PMC1274154/?page=2

(15) Frisch, R. E. (1987, August). Body fat, menarche, fitness and fertility. Retrieved from https://www.ncbi.nlm.nih.gov/pubmed/3117838

(16) Types of Fat. (2018, July 24). Retrieved from https://www.hsph.harvard.edu/nutritionsource/what-should-you-eat/fats-and-cholesterol/types-of-fat/

(17) Barnard, N. D., Bunner, A. E., & Agarwal, U. (2014, May 15) Saturated and trans fats and dementia: A systematic review Retrieved   from https://www.sciencedirect.com/science/article/pii/S019745801 4003558

(18) Tuso, P., Stoll, S. R., & Li, W. W. (2015). A Plant-Based Diet, Atherogenesis, and Coronary Artery Disease Prevention Retrieved   from https://www.ncbi.nlm.nih.gov/pmc/articles/PMC4315380/

(19) . Targeting Insulin Resistance: The Ongoing Paradigm Shift in Diabetes Prevention. American Journal of Managed Care April 11, 2013. http://www.ajmc.com/journals/evidence-based-diabetes-management/2013/2013-1-vol19-sp2/targeting-insulin-resistance-the-ongoing-paradigm-shift-in-diabetes-prevention

(20) National Institute of Diabetes, Digestive and Kidney Diseases: Prediabetes and Insulin Resistance. August 9 2009. https://www.niddk.nih.gov/healthinformation/diabetes/ types/prediabetes-insulin-resistance

(21) Orgel: The Links Between Insulin Resistance, Diabetes, and Cancer. Curr Diab Rep. 2013 Apr; 13(2): 213–222 https://www.ncbi.nlm.nih.gov/pmc/articles/PMC3595327/

(22) Mozaffari-Khosravi, H., Yassini-Ardakani, M., Karamati M., & Shariati-Bafghi, S. E. (2013, July). Eicosapentaenoic acid versus docosahexaenoic acid in mild-to-moderate depression: A randomized, double-blind, placebo-controlled trial. Retrieved from https://www.ncbi.nlm.nih.gov/pubmed/22910528

(23) Types of Fat. (2018, July 24). Retrieved from https://www.hsph.harvard.edu/nutritionsource/what-should-you-eat/fats-and-cholesterol/types-of-fat/

(24) D. (n.d.). Trans Fats. Retrieved from https://www.dietitians.ca/Dietitians-Views/Food-Regulation-and-Labelling/Trans-Fats.aspx

(25) University of Utah, N. (n.d.). Food Storage and Nutrients. Retrieved from http://www3.uakron.edu/chima/text/Food storage article 8-05.pdf

(26) Bidlingmaier, M., & Strasburger, C. J. (n.d.). Growth hormone. Retrieved from https://www.ncbi.nlm.nih.gov/pubmed/20020365

(27) Bidlingmaier, M., & Strasburger, C. J. (n.d.). Growth hormone. Retrieved from https://www.ncbi.nlm.nih.gov/pubmed/20020365

(28) Blackman, M. R., Sorkin, J. D., Münzer, T., Bellantoni, M. F., Busby-Whitehead, J., Stevens, T. E., . . . Harman, S. M. (2002, November 13). Growth hormone and sex steroid administration in healthy aged women and men: A randomized controlled trial. Retrieved from https://www.ncbi.nlm.nih.gov/pubmed/12425705

(29) Ho, K. Y., Veldhuis, J. D., Johnson, M. L., Furlanetto, R., Evans, W. S., Alberti, K. G., & Thorner, M. O. (1988, April). Fasting enhances growth hormone secretion and amplifies the complex rhythms of growth hormone secretion. Retrieved from https://www.ncbi.nlm.nih.gov/pmc/articles/PMC329619/

(30) Varady, K. A., Bhutani, S., Klempel, M. C., Kroeger, C. M., Trepanowski, J. F., Haus, J. M., . . . Calvo, Y. (2013). Alternate day fasting for weight loss in normal weight and overweight subjects: A randomized controlled trial. Retrieved from https://www.ncbi.nlm.nih.gov/pmc/articles/PMC3833266/

(31) Schwartz, J., & Gladding, R. (2012). *You are not your brain: The 4-step solution for changing bad habits, ending unhealthy thinking, and taking control of your life.* New York: Penguin Group.

(32) Locke, E. A., & Shaw, K. (n.d.). Goal Setting and Task Performance. Retrieved from http://www.dtic.mil/dtic/tr/fulltext/u2/a086584.pdf

(33) Fasting and the risk of dehydration during Ramadan. (n.d.). Retrieved from https://www.hamad.qa/EN/your health/Ramadan Health/Health Information/Pages/Dehydration.aspx

(34) Rogers, K. (2016, April 07). Trans fat. Retrieved from https://www.britannica.com/science/trans-fat

(35) Harland, B. F. (n.d.). Caffeine and nutrition. Retrieved from https://www.nutritionjrnl.com/article/S0899-9007(00)00369-5/abstract

Check out other Books by Jamie Connor

Meal Prep – Ultimate Guide

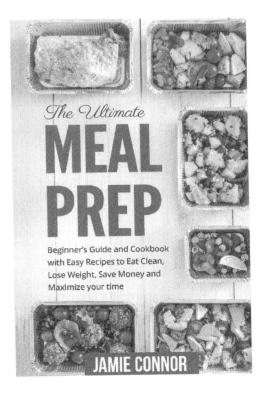

One Final Thing...

Did You Enjoy and Find This Book Useful?

If you did, please let me know by leaving a review on AMAZON Reviews lets Amazon knows that I am providing quality material to my readers. Even a few words and rating would go a long way. I would like to thank you in advance for your time.

If you didn't, please shoot me an email at jamieconnor@bmccpublishing.com and let me know what you didn't like. I maybe able to change or update it.

Lastly, if you have any feedback to improve the book, please email me. In this age, this book can be a living book. It can be continuously improved by feedback provided by readers like you.

About The Author

Jamie Connor is a certified personal trainer, yoga instructor, and nutrition coach that currently lives in Miami Florida. After graduating from Cornell University with a Ms in Nutrition, Jamie is currently working for a Fortune 500 company in Miami. Growing up in a family that consumed a lot of process foods, Jamie struggled with obesity and health problems. After almost losing her life 6 years ago, Jamie made a decision to develop a healthy lifestyle. When Jamie started exercising and eliminating processed foods from her diet, things started to turn around. She felt stronger and energy levels were through the roof.

Today, Jamie is on a mission to share what she had learned with her readers to get the same results. In addition, through multiple trial and errors, she developed many healthy and delicious recipes that are full of flavor, texture and wholesome nutrition.

Jamie also enjoys practicing yoga, reading, and traveling around the world to discover new recipes.

32881250R00099

Made in the USA
Middletown, DE
08 January 2019